NOTE TO USERS

This information is considered by B.C. Cancer Agency staff to offer clear, general information concerning cancer care which will help to answer frequently asked questions. However, in some instances, it may contain treatment or related information which varies from Agency practice.

This material is not intended to replace advice given by your physician or other health care providers. If you have any questions or would like more current information or further guidance, you are encouraged to speak to your cancer specialist, other Clinic staff or your personal physician.

The selections from *Aesop's Fables* are used by permission of Grosset & Dunlap, Inc.

"The Magic Word," page 89, and "The Fruit," page 210, are from Idries Shah, *The Dermis Probe*. They are used by permission of Curtis Brown, Ltd. and Jonathan Cape Ltd.

"The Idiot, the Wise Man, and the Jug," page 77, and "The Tale of the Sands," page 120, are from *Tales of the Dervishes*, by Idries Shah. They are used by permission of E.P. Dutton & Co., Inc. and Curtis Brown, Ltd.

Library of Congress Catalog Number: 78-4529

Original Prentice-Hall edition published in 1978,
ISBN 0-13-314021-0 clothbound
ISBN 0-13-314013-X paperbound

New, updated Celestial Arts edition First Printing 1986,
ISBN 0-89087-458-1

Celestial Arts
P.O. Box 7327
Berkeley, California 94707

Cover Design by Ken Scott

Made in the United States of America

10 9 8 7 6 5 4 3   — 90 89 88

To my mother, Harryette Barton,
whose faith and love
have shone like a beacon
through my life

NOTE TO USERS

This information is considered by B.C. Cancer Agency staff to offer clear, general information concerning cancer care which will help to answer frequently asked questions. However, in some instances, it may contain treatment or related information which varies from Agency practice.

This material is not intended to replace advice given by your physician or other health care providers. If you have any questions or would like more current information or further guidance, you are encouraged to speak to your cancer specialist, other Clinic staff or your personal physician.

Man alone, of all the creatures of earth, can change his own pattern. Man alone is architect of his destiny. The greatest revolution in our generation is the discovery that human beings, by changing the inner attitudes of their minds, can change the outer aspects of their lives.

WILLIAM JAMES

Foreword

by Ken Pelletier, Ph.D.
Assistant Clinical Professor,
Dept. of Medicine,
University of California, San Francisco

For the last decade, Dr. Miller and I have traveled along similar professional paths in our explorations of the mind-body relationship. Originally we and our fellow explorers were viewed with some skepticism, both by the medical establishment and the general population. Now we find ourselves among an extraordinary company of researchers, health practitioners, and business leaders promoting a new approach to health care in which *all* the determinants of disease—physical, social, psychological, environmental, and spiritual—are considered.

Today there is a growing awareness that it makes more sense to prevent disease than to wait for symptoms. The economic costs of ignoring this simple fact have become intolerable for our society; great changes are taking place all around us. Even beyond dealing with what we've always known as illness, there is a realization that we can expect more of ourselves than just keeping out of the doctor's office. People recognize that there are degrees of health as well as degrees of illness, and they want to know *how* they can reach their own optimal level of health, performance, and life fulfillment. This book helps to answer that question. The need is great, the response is timely.

Dr. Miller's book represents a cornerstone in thinking about the human being, and about how an individual's self-image can be used to influence health. Scientific research confirms that this relationship exists on the deepest biological levels, in the brain and in the immune system. It has become very clear that the way we perceive ourselves has a profound influence on physiological processes. These are exciting times indeed, as we see more and more clearly that we are not the passive victims of our fate, but can exert control and change our selves, both figuratively and literally.

Most importantly, the new health message is one of hope and personal responsibility. It's also one of good humor; we can be serious about health and illness without being somber, and you can look forward to a book that is not only educational but also enjoyable. This is an important work which demonstrates new ways to see yourself and guide you into your own empowerment.

Contents

Preface
and
acknowledgments

In the early part of the 1970's, while engaged in the practice of Family Medicine, I found myself feeling profoundly frustrated and disappointed. Although my medical training had been one of the finest available in the world, I found myself unable to treat adequately the overwhelming majority of diseases that I encountered on a daily basis.

Of course I could prescribe pain killers, muscle relaxants, tranquilizers and the other symptomatic remedies that make up the majority of the drugs that physicians prescribe, but unlike many of my colleagues at the time I could not ignore the facts that stared me in the face. Even though the symptom was relieved, it was only temporarily, the drugs often had unpleasant side effects, and a certain "glow of health" did not return to the cheeks of my patients.

Their problems—back pain, high blood pressure, fatigue, overweight, smoking, cancer, and the like—were primarily the result of poor stress management, faulty lifestyle and self care habits, inadequate exercise and sleep, and other factors that I had no way to influence. How I longed for a nice, clearcut case of malaria, or tuberculosis—something my tools equipped me to deal with. As a result, I found myself searching for means by which I could empower people to change their attitudes and their lives, ways to put people in charge of their own bodies and behaviors.

Preface and Acknowledgments

One of my earliest discoveries occurred at a social gathering of physicians. I heard a highly esteemed colleague discussing how he had successfully treated a patient who suffered acute muscular spasm of the back by using hypnotherapy. Dubious at first, I asked for more information and attended a few weekend seminars on Medical Hypnosis. Impressed with what I had seen, I began to use these techniques in my work and to explore other fields, such as meditation, biofeedback, autogenic training, and behavior therapy.

Before long, my experiences crystallized. I realized that it was possible for people to eliminate painful physical symptoms and diseases and to produce dramatic changes in their health and in the quality of their lives by learning simple tools of relaxation and imagery.

After years of practicing medicine and working in hospitals, I had vivid memories of women screaming for hours in the labor room, of patients suffering from serious complications after surgery, of cancer victims requiring round-the-clock narcotics to free them from their agony. There were young and old alike who would stay home and put up with painful symptoms rather than face their fears of doctors, hospitalization, and surgery; and there were hypertension patients tied to drugs for a lifetime and constantly threatened by the fear of a serious heart attack, and many more . . . . And here were simple techniques that could resolve many of these problems! Rather than being forced to be dependent on medication or doctors, I realized that patients could be taught to control their own health and well-being.

As they were when I found them, each of these fields had its strengths, but the weaknesses of each were severe. And not the least of these weaknesses was that each seemed vehemently to deny the efficacy of the others. To me, however, the similarities were obvious, and for several years I strove to integrate them into a single, effective, scientifically sound system. As a name for this system I chose the most important single tool for self change, *Selective Awareness.*

Selective Awareness is a wellness tool because, unlike traditional medical techniques it provides tools that you can apply in your own life to maintain physical, mental, and emotional health. By health I mean two things—that the physiological processes within your body are in *dynamic balance,* and, equally important, that you *feel good!*

With the techniques you will learn in this book, the control and responsibility for your health is in your hands, not in the hands of a doctor or therapist. The doctor is a valuable expert consultant, but it is up to you to decide when you need this consultation, and whether or not you choose to follow the advice given. The ultimate responsibility is yours, whether you choose to recognize it or not.

In this book I present the techniques gradually so you can begin to understand how the human mind creates the conditions for disease to develop. I've included many case studies of people who have been able to resolve their problems by learning these processes. You'll have an opportunity to clarify your own attitudes on health and healing.

If you are suffering from a painful or uncomfortable physical symptom, emotional problem, or troublesome habit that you'd like to be free of; if you would like to learn some practical information about dealing with the tension and stresses in everyday life; and enjoying your leisure time more fully—then this book is for you.

In addition to learning how you can cope more effectively with medications and surgery when they are necessary, and the discomfort caused by painful physical symptoms and disease, you will see how you can begin to change your attitudes about health. In each of us lies the natural tendency toward physical health, psychological satisfaction, and creativity. You'll learn how to discover these natural tools within yourself and use them for your benefit in everyday life.

Some of the case studies will be startling. You will see how chronic problems of stomach and intestinal pain, muscle-spasm, and ulcers have been resolved. People with long histories of allergies, hay fever, and repeated colds have put an end to these patterns. Problems of chronic depression, continuous anxiety, pounding heart, sweaty palms, high blood pressure, sexual problems, and such habits as overeat-

ing and smoking have been eliminated. Even tremors, hypo-
gylcemia, migraine headaches, backaches, and visual problems have dramatically improved.

I have seen people change their lives through the use of
these processes. My purpose in writing this book is to open
the door for you to discover these tools. You no longer need
to remain the victim of your physical and emotional problems. With a responsible attitude and motivation, you also
can dramatically change your life.

Those to whom I owe the most gratitude for help in
creating this book can not be mentioned by name. When I
relate their stories, their names are changed, and even the
details are changed slightly in order to further protect their
identities. They are the patients, clients, and students whose
willingness to trust in themselves has made possible all the
pages to follow.

A very special thanks is due to Deborah Leuth who
worked closely with me in the process of assembling and or-
ganizing and converting into readable English an almost infi-
nite pile of facts, observations, experiences, and case histories. I imagine that I might have had to work twice as hard in
the preparation of Chapter 5 had it not been for Ken Pelletier whose painstaking research for his book *Mind As Healer,
Mind As Slayer* provided the opportunity for me to link my
work and its results with that of other clinicians and investigators around the world.

Most people are aware of how vital moral support is to
an athlete to avoid becoming "psyched out." Writers, I have
found, are prone to the same hazard. Support in my days of
sagging spirit came from Jim Fadiman, Ph.D., who also
helped me locate a publisher for this work, as well as from
Russel Wills, Ph.D. and Arthur Hastings, Ph.D., who also
helped in assembling the material. Nor do I want to forget
Marleen Olds and Jackie Wood, whose help was most valuable in getting the manuscript into its final form.

E.E.M.

Introduction

In each of us lies the natural ability to keep ourselves healthy and satisfied. Why, then, must we use tranquilizers, muscle relaxants, and sleeping pills to relieve headaches, aching muscles, high blood pressure, indigestion, ulcers, and sleepless nights?

As the twentieth century draws to a close, an important new concept has entered the field of medicine. It is the idea of patient-centered medicine, of self care, of *wellness,* in which individuals recognize and accept personal responsibility for their own health and rediscover their own natural healing abilities. In our society, only a hermit could fail to notice this change. We are moving away from inappropriate dependence on drugs and doctors and towards empowerment. We are seeing that we can be in control of our own health.

This approach has also been described as holistic, or integral medicine, reflecting a focus on the whole person rather than on isolated parts and symptoms. It is also known as humanistic medicine, describing the development of full human potential by strengthening the part that is well rather than attacking the part that is not. Wellness medicine sees physical, mental, and emotional problems as inevitably linked together. Its goal is the resolution of these problems.

An important key to achieving this goal is your own motivation. Learning how to allow your natural health-restoring abilities to work for you is like learning to ride a bicycle — a bit clumsy and awkward at first, trying to coordinate arms, legs, and balance. But motivation keeps you working at it, and soon you're relaxed and expert, riding effortlessly and automatically. And as everyone knows, once you learn, you never forget!

Awakening your natural potential for self healing and wellness requires that a change take place — not one that is forced upon you by medication or surgery, but one that you must consciously desire and initiate in yourself. It begins with a change in how you think and feel, and in the perspective from which you view yourself and your environment. The first step in accepting new structures and patterns of this kind is to be open to exploring new possibilities. This is accomplished through the process of imagination — the willful suspension of disbelief.

We do this when someone tells us a joke, and we did it as children when we read a fairy tale. But freedom of creativity and imagination tend to diminish as we leave childhood and grow older, along with the ability to learn new skills. Encouraged by social norms, adults restrict themselves to figuring things out, rationalizing, and explaining. For total wellness we must each build an internal environment in which learning takes place through *creative experiences* as well as *rational thought*.

The purpose of this book is to familiarize you with what is often called "the new medicine," and in particular to introduce you to your own capacity to achieve selective awareness and move towards your optimum state of health. The state of mind involved—openmindedness—is similar to that involved in reading a story or hearing a joke, and I have included some time-honored stories and fables to help describe the principles involved.

There are also case histories about people who have let their own healing abilities work for them. You will see how they have alleviated symptoms arising from physical or emotional problems, or from negative habits, by getting to their roots. You will gain a clear picture of how tension and stress can create disease, and how you can control them. You will then see some applications of these principles in medicine, education, and psychotherapy.

As you read, you may notice similarities between these approaches and guided imagery, autogenic training, yoga, prayer, and hypnosis. All of these have many features in common. They use relaxation, suggestion, and imagery and require repeated application. They also have important differences. Though the processes we will examine had their root in hypnotherapy, the most important factor here is that the people seeking help learn tools that they can apply in their lives to maintain physical and emotional health and well-being. They remain awake and alert throughout the process and remember all that occurs; there are no mystical or magical words, symbols, or phrases. The control of, and responsibility for, the person is ultimately in his or her own hands—*not* in the hands of the doctor or therapist. This book is the result of years of observing these phenomena working in thousands of people. These observations have led to clarification of principles that can help you to explore and expand your abilities to heal yourself and maintain health.

Until quite recently, hypnosis has been discussed in medical schools only from a historical perspective. Even now, techniques and practical applications are just beginning to be taught. Now, an increasing number of physicians, nurses, dentists, psychologists, psychiatrists, and surgeons have become interested in the tools of hypnosis. Physicians and scientists are now beginning to study hypnosis and its value in promoting health and healing. Hypnotic procedures are being applied in maternity care, cardiac care, cancer therapy, oral surgery, and other areas.

The use of modern hypnotic and meditative methods has strong implications for medicine and psychology. One of the central concerns in all physical symptoms, diseases, or unwanted habit patterns is *pain* — physical pain or psychological pain. The sensation of pain can temporarily bring to a halt all ordinary activities, habits, routines, problems, and emotions such as anger, joy, depression, or fear. If you step on a nail, all your thoughts, feelings, sensations, and perceptions immediately become irrelevant. For a few moments, everything else is blocked but the experience of pain. In the hypnotic state, pain can be reduced through the use of the body's natural mechanisms with complete self control. If we can eliminate this powerful sensation of pain in the hypnotic state, it follows that we can also use it to create temporary freedom and relief from unwanted physical symptoms, habits, and emotional patterns. In the relaxed state we can then focus on the underlying roots of problems, understand them, and probably eliminate them forever.

The key components of the processes described in this book are *deep relaxation, self awareness,* and *imagery.* The techniques for achieving these three are derived from numerous clinical disciplines, including biofeedback, autogenic training, meditation, hypnotherapy, and behavioral medicine. They will enable you to achieve alert, focused attention in a state of deep relaxation. I have named this state *selective awareness,* and it can be a powerful healing tool for you.

I

A new plan for health

The cat and the fox

A fox was boasting to a cat one day about how clever he was. "Why, I have a whole bag of tricks," he bragged. "For instance, I know of at least a hundred different ways of escaping my enemies, the dogs."

"How remarkable," said the cat. "As for me, I have only one trick, though I usually make it work. I wish you could teach me some of yours."

"Well, sometime when I have nothing else to do," said the fox, "I might teach you one or two of my easier ones."

Just at that moment they heard the yelping of a pack of hounds. They were coming straight toward the spot where the cat and the fox stood. Like a flash the cat scampered up a tree and disappeared in the foliage. "This is the trick I told you about," she called down to the fox. "It's my only one. Which trick are you going to use?"

The fox sat there trying to decide which of his many tricks he was going to employ. Nearer and nearer came the hounds. When it was quite too late, the fox decided to run for it. But even before he started the dogs were upon him, and that was the end of the fox, bagful of tricks and all!

APPLICATION: One good plan that works is better than a hundred doubtful ones.

Introduction to part I

In the first section of the book, we'll begin to build a framework in which to understand health and nonhealth, or disease. In Chapter 1, we'll discuss exactly what we mean by "health," both in terms of physical balance and psychological well-being. You'll be able to observe how tension and anxiety are key components of disease.

We'll explore the vast potential of the human mind and how we can master some of this potential and bring it into the realm of everyday life. Relaxation and its effects on the mind and body will be a central tool that we'll explore; in Chapter 2 you'll see how it can be used to control stress and tension.

In Chapter 3, we'll explore how emotions affect physical health and how the two are inextricably linked. In Chapter 4, tension and anxiety will be discussed in detail. We've included case studies of people with the most common physical ailments in our culture to give you a broad view of how relaxation can be an effective tool in treating painful physical symptoms.

In Chapter 5, we'll review some of the major research

of the last decade that demonstrates the importance of unifying the mind and body in healing. Treating the mind and body as one integrated, functioning unit leads to a new view of medical science. Practitioners of this "new medicine" report that their clients experience dramatic changes in the quality of their lives—new attitudes, new goals, new motivations—leading to increased satisfaction and well-being.

We will conclude Part I with a brief view of medical science as it is practiced in our culture. The material covered in Chapter 6 will be covered more extensively in Part III.

In reading Part I, pay attention to your own attitudes and experiences. What does health mean to you? Do you fully and completely enjoy your leisure time? Do you carry unnecessary tension with you through the day? Which mental, physical, and emotional ailments and diseases can you relieve? How often do you go to a doctor? And most important, how is your health right now—*at this moment*? Do you *feel good*?

1
Balance and health

The oak and the reed

A proud oak grew upon the bank of a stream. For a full hundred years it had withstood the buffeting of the winds, but one day there came a violent storm. The great oak fell with a mighty crash into the swollen river and was carried down toward the sea.

Later the oak tree came to rest on the shore where some reeds were growing. The tree was amazed to see the reeds standing upright.

"How ever did you manage to weather that terrible storm?" he asked. "I have stood up against many a storm, but this one was too strong for me."

"That's just it," replied the reed. "All these years you have stubbornly pitted your great strength against the wind. You were too proud to yield a little. I, on the other hand, knowing my weakness, just bend and let the wind blow over me without trying

to resist it. The harder the wind blows the more I humble myself, so here I am!"

APPLICATION: It is better to bend than to break.

Our bodies are continually in a state of flux. Physiological *balance* is maintained by the buildup of new cells and the destruction of old ones, the alternate tension and relaxation of muscles, and the constant influx and outflow of intercellular fluids, water and dissolved gases. This balance, the tendency of the body to maintain a state of equilibrium, is called *homeostasis* and is a most important part of the condition we refer to as *health*.

We can also describe *balance* in terms of our feelings. Imagine yourself waking up early one morning. The morning air is fresh, and you lie in bed comfortably for a few minutes, stretching and taking a few deep breaths. You notice how good it feels to have slept well, and you're ready to start the day. It's a work day, and you're aware of a long list of things that need to be done. You know the day will be busy, and you'll have to be efficient in order to meet your obligations; but you feel good about it—you're alert and energetic. You feel as though things will turn out well; you'll take one task at a time and enjoy the satisfaction of doing a good job.

Now the day is over; you're tired but not tense. You've worked hard today and feel satisfied. You can put the day's task aside and enjoy dinner, reading, stimulating exercise, dancing, an evening with your family or friends, or whatever activity you choose. As the evening gets late, you notice yourself becoming more and more relaxed, and you go to bed and fall asleep feeling comfortable and content.

We would describe this situation by saying that you are functioning in a state of *balance*: You sleep comfortably and naturally, feel energetic and satisfied, and can relax and enjoy yourself after a difficult day; in other words, you *feel good*. In a state of natural health, the body maintains a continual state of physical, mental, and emotional balance. All too often, however, we may find ourselves in a state of imbalance. Physiological imbalance occurs when there is too much buildup or breakdown of body cells or cellular structures, too much tension in the muscles, or when the normal flux of cellular fluids and gases is interrupted. We often call the state of imbalance *disease.*

We can also look at imbalance in relationship to our feelings. We might call it "getting up on the wrong side of the bed." A mother may watch her child running through the house with muddy shoes and get a headache; a businessman may come home with indigestion after spending eight stressful hours at a desk; a student who is angry with his or her professor may notice tension in the neck and shoulders; a musician may get diarrhea before an important performance. We can all recognize the feelings that accompany imbalance—frustration, discouragement, unhappiness, confusion, depression, fear, anger, and so on. If these physical symptoms and their emotional counterparts continue, the housewife may end up with regular migraine headaches: the businessman, with an ulcer; the student, with severe muscle spasm; and the musician, with colitis, which may make it impossible for him to perform at all. *Imbalance can create changes in the body and cause physical symptoms*. This imbalance, then, is at the root of physical changes we refer to as *disease*. Healing is the process by which the organism returns to its functional state of balance—health.

An imbalance (emotional, mental, or physical) may be present for some time before the physical *symptoms* become severe enough to attract our attention. For example, the symptoms of a cold or the flu are often preceded by a general tension in the body, tiredness, and feelings of anxiety, which are the cues to an imbalance. If we have learned the importance of paying attention to these cues and understand the link between emotional states and physical symptoms, we can give our body the relaxation, rest, and relief it is asking for and perhaps avoid the onset of a sore throat, cough, or headache that could easily require much more time to heal. Let us now begin to look at how our natural healing potential can work to keep us healthy.

Adaptive tension and maladaptive tension

It has become very fashionable to talk about relaxation. Nearly every popular journal carries articles on how to "sit back and relax!" It would almost appear that the ideal body is like a wet noodle, lethargically slumping over every available chair or leaning post.

It is necessary for the body, in its natural state of flux, to maintain certain levels of tension that allow an appropriate response to the environment. This is called *tonus*, or tone. Let's look at an example of balance in which the body functions effectively and *adaptively* in a state of tension followed by a natural state of relaxation.

Imagine a situation where you see a small child running into the street unaware of a rapidly approaching car. Though you may not notice it, there is an increase in your heartbeat and breathing and accompanying feelings you might identify as fear, tension, and anxiety. This tension causes the central nervous system to send sympathetic hormones such as adrenalin through your vascular system so you can move swiftly and effectively to handle the situation. After the child is safely out of danger, the internal alarm quiets, and your body gradually calms down, leaving you feeling relaxed and relieved. There is a moment or two of profound relaxation as you "heave a sigh of relief." Oxygen and energy supplies are replenished, and your body returns to its normal resting balance.

We are all familiar with this type of tension—it's an *adaptive* response that allows us to cope with our environment in the most efficient way. In this way, the body functions in a state of dynamic balance—the rise and subsequent fall in physical tension and emotional anxiety.

Imbalance occurs when we retain a level of tension in our bodies and a level of emotional anxiety that is *maladaptive*, i.e., tension and anxiety that do not help us in coping with our environment. A high degree of tension before giving an important speech, before an important interview, or before going to bed can be maladaptive. We may experience nervousness, anxiety, restlessness, frustration, and depression as we struggle against the unwanted tension. Before long we may find ourselves with headaches, ulcers, or the symptoms of heart disease.

The following criteria are helpful in determining whether or not a specific physical sensation, emotion, or habit pattern is *maladaptive*:

1. It is unpleasant to know you have this pattern.

2. It is not useful (your life would run more smoothly without it).

3. Sometimes it is harmful and decreases your ability to cope with your environment and feel satisfied.

4. You would be happier without it.

5. You have no need for it; you would like to control it in future situations rather than have it control you.

6. It is often associated with a general feeling of tension.

The usual remedies for unwanted mental and physical tension include tranquilizers, muscle relaxants, aspirin, sleeping pills, or simply "putting up with it" and learning to ignore it. You may get used to having asthma every spring, headaches every time you have a stressful day, painful menstrual cramps every month, or sleepless nights. You find yourself describing how you feel or how parts of your body feel as "not so bad" or as having various degrees of discomfort. You may even forget how it feels to wake up in the morning feeling refreshed, energetic, and excited about new challenges—you may forget what it's like to really *feel good*. You may begin to enjoy your work, your school, your family, or your leisure time less and less while feeling anxious and discouraged more and more. It becomes a vicious cycle, and suddenly you may find yourself with serious physical problems. You may ask, "What happened to the natural healing abilities that are supposed to maintain a state of balance?" Most of us have never learned what they are or how to use them. Just as we can't build a shelf if we leave the hammer in the tool box, we can't use our healing potential if it is stored away.

> A medieval cathedral was being built, and three stonecutters were asked in turn, "What are you doing?" The first replied in an angry tone, "As you see, I am cutting stones."

The second answered, "I am earning a living for myself and my family." And the third said joyously, "I am building a great cathedral!" Each was doing the same task of cutting the stones, one with a sense of boredom and futility, one with a personal purpose, and one with true understanding. He knew that each stone he cut was important to the building of the beautiful cathedral.

We will use the concept of balance in the next chapters as a reference in describing how we can begin to "build" our health and begin to use our natural tools. Imagine that you are much like the third stonecutter, aware that each step you take toward learning how to control your own health, no matter how small, is equally important. Enjoy each step *now* and you will have joyous benefits later!

The conscious mind and the nonconscious mind

At any moment we can talk about two parts of ourselves. For our purposes, we will call them the *conscious* mind and the *nonconscious* mind.[1] When thoughts and feelings are brought into your present awareness (become aware of the page you are reading, your immediate surroundings, the clothes you are wearing), we call them *conscious*. The conscious mind has limited storage facilities and handles information one or two pieces at a time. This can easily be demonstrated by a short experiment:

Become aware of your middle name. Now become aware of the sole of your left foot. Become aware of the town in

---

[1]Due to the many different interpretations of "unconscious" and "subconscious," we will use the term *nonconscious* to mean simply that which is not in one's *conscious* awareness.

which you were born, your telephone number, and now your favorite food. Now become aware of all these things simultaneously!

You can see the difficulty of being aware of many things at one time. It's easy to demonstrate how easily the conscious mind "overloads" and becomes confused and disorganized. On the other hand, its ability to retrieve specific details is extraordinary. You are able to focus acutely and clearly on a specific memory in your life, one of millions, by simply desiring to do so.

The conscious mind can focus attention so acutely that other incoming stimuli may be temporarily blocked. While involved in an active sport, have you ever sustained a minor injury such as a cut, bruise, or scrape and not been aware of it? Your focus on the activity may have completely blocked the sensation of pain from that area. Your first awareness that you had been injured might have been minutes or hours later when a friend pointed to the area and asked what happened. At this moment you become aware of the discomfort, which might have served later that same night to keep you awake for hours. Had your mind been less focused on your participation in the sport, you might have noticed the discomfort at the time of the injury. Athletes have been known to play an entire football game ignorant of the fact that they had fractured a rib during the first quarter. The impulses never reached the conscious mind, because they were blocked by the concentration and excitement produced by focusing on the game.

The nonconscious mind

The nonconscious mind and its functions are fascinating. It has exceptional storage capacities and handles large quantities of information. The nonconscious holds the record of your life experiences. Thoughts that can easily be brought to conscious awareness are stored in the nonconscious. This includes old addresses, names of high school teachers, where you were last Friday night, and so on and on. Thoughts that seem to defy being brought into consciousness or thoughts that seem temporarily irretrievable are also stored here. This would include a misplaced object or a "forgotten" name. There are also many thoughts stored in the nonconscious that you will probably never recall at all such as many childhood memories. Finally, the functions of your autonomic nervous system are included in the nonconscious: the change in your pupil size when you walk from the darkness into bright sunlight, the change in your heartbeat when you are jogging, the change in blood flow to your hands and feet when you are nervous, the tension and restlessness you feel when your muscles have not been exercised for some time, and the stomach contractions that cause you to feel hungry when your body needs food.

The following common situation demonstrates the storage capacity of the nonconscious mind:

Imagine entering your bedroom, living room, or office. As you walk in the door and scan the familiar scene, you are likely to notice a magazine on the floor, a vase out of place on the end table, a plant that is turned in a different direction than when you left, or a pen in an unusual position on your desk. Anything out of the ordinary attracts your attention immediately. Your mind and your eyes have taken in literally thousands of stimuli, yet a single element out of place will be instantly noted by the nonconscious mind "automatically" and brought into your conscious awareness for consideration. You can tell immediately that something has changed in the room since you left it.

You can imagine the extremely complicated list that

would be necessary to enable a person to make similar discoveries if he or she were unfamiliar with the room. Checking a written list as accurate as your memory might take hours to reveal what your mind sees instantaneously. During a split second, your mind can perform all these activities, inspecting each of the individual items and comparing them with previously stored information about the room. All this can be performed with as little effort as recalling your name.

If we want to understand a disease and its physical and emotional components, we must look at the nonconscious mind. Of course, we don't choose our health problems and diseases consciously. It is in the nonconscious, the vast storehouse of our life experience, that we find the clues to our problems and the roots of the disease.

2
Relaxation

The hare and the tortoise

A hare was continually poking fun at a tortoise because of the slowness of his pace. The tortoise tried not to be annoyed by the jeers of the hare, but one day in the presence of the other animals he was goaded into challenging the hare to a foot race.

"Why, this a joke," said the hare. "You know that I can run circles around you."

"Enough of your boasting," said the tortoise. "Let's get on with the race."

So the course was set by the animals, and the fox was chosen as judge. He gave a sharp bark and the race was on. Almost before you could say "scat" the hare was out of sight. The tortoise plodded along at his usual unhurried pace.

After a time the hare stopped to wait for the tortoise to come along. He waited for a long, long time until he began to get sleepy. "I'll just take a quick nap here in this soft grass, and then in the

19

cool of the day I'll finish the race." So he lay down and closed his eyes.

Meanwhile, the tortoise plodded on. He passed the sleeping hare, and was approaching the finish line when the hare awoke with a start. It was too late to save the race. Much ashamed, he crept away while all the animals at the finish line acclaimed the winner.

APPLICATION: Slow and steady wins the race.

We are all familiar with the feelings associated with relaxation. Most of us, however, are unaware of how to relax ourselves voluntarily during periods of stress. In the last decade, more and more evidence has been accumulated to demonstrate that natural relaxation is necessary to the maintenance of health and balance. By learning to relax, we can begin to eliminate the symptoms caused or made worse by physical and emotional tension. Tension and anxiety are important components of ninety percent or more of the medical problems most familiar to us!

Descriptions of "relaxation" will vary from individual to individual and within the same individual from time to time. Your idea of a *relaxing* day might include walking on the beach, lying in the sun, and enjoying a good book. Your closest friend might find the beach undesirable and much prefer to relax by taking a cable car ride or going on a hike to a mountain lake surrounded by beautiful pines. Likewise, notions of "pleasant" or "relaxing" music vary from one person to another.

Imagine the feeling of awakening in the morning. This morning begins a weekend or a holiday, and there is no work ahead. The sun is shining in on you, and you awake slowly. Before you open your eyes, you can feel yourself comfortably floating, almost as though your body were enveloped in a cloud. Your imagination is vivid and creative. Dream characters cavort in the misty borders of your mind. As you open your eyes and become more and more awake, you begin to feel the "real world" gently tumble in on you. You become aware of your surroundings, the time, and you begin to think about getting up. In this state of relaxation you feel comfortable, calm, content.

The somewhat faraway feeling you experience just before opening your eyes in the morning is similar to being "lost in thought." On such an occasion someone may notice that you have a glassy look in your eyes and that you seem to be staring off into space; they may ask you what you're thinking about. The question might startle you, and you might respond by saying, "Oh, I was just daydreaming." Your mind was focusing on your internal thoughts and images.

Inherent in the state of relaxation is the ability to acutely focus awareness and attention. If the focus is on internal thoughts, the imagination becomes active and vivid. Perhaps you can remember being so engrossed in a book that you didn't hear someone calling your name though they were standing only a few feet away. So interested were you in what you were reading that it absorbed your complete attention. Compare this state of relaxed awareness with the tense concentration you may have experienced when studying for a difficult examination. Even the slightest sound may become an annoying distraction.

It's easy to see that learning to relax involves no work; it's rather like learning *not to work*. This may be a difficult task for those of us who have grown up with the notion that we should always be *doing* something. Many of us are so accustomed to judging and evaluating ourselves that relaxing becomes a "task." Relaxation is actually the *passive* concentration of the mind that ensues when we abandon the task of remaining acutely aware of the external environment and problems connected with it. Spontaneous thoughts from the nonconscious can then pass through to awareness unhindered. Such relaxation is often described as *comfortable, calm, warm, gentle, pleasant, feeling good*. Being relaxed is one way in which we can be in balance and let our natural healing processes emerge, as we will observe. Each of you might describe your feeling of relaxation a little differently; yet you'll no doubt agree that it's something you'd like to experience more often!

The process of natural relaxation

Relaxation occurs with the accumulation of relaxing thoughts, feelings, and body sensations. Many of you may be more familiar with the opposite condition: tension. Tension occurs with the accumulation of stressful thoughts, anxious feelings, and muscular tightness. Imagine how this situation might occur:

You are driving home from work, from school, or from an afternoon errand. You've had a good day and are looking forward to an evening with your family or friends. On the way home you remember a letter that you need to mail today, and you quickly change direction so you can get to the post office before it closes. It seems as though all the traffic lights are against you—each one turns red just before you get to the intersection. You begin glancing at your watch every couple of minutes. The traffic is getting heavier; and a car is stalled up ahead, so one of the lanes is closed. You find yourself creeping along slowly in the midst of heavy traffic, and you know you can't make it to the post office on time! As you start home again, you think, "All this extra driving for nothing!" You finally arrive home an hour late and sink into a chair, frustrated and discouraged.

What happened? Each new thought that enters the mind builds on all the ones previously stored there. Any related series of thoughts creates a rhythm in the mind. As momentum is built, a train of thoughts tends to maintain itself without additional energy just as your foot keeps tapping or you keep on singing just after listening to a catchy tune. This is similar to the spinning of a top—once the top reaches a certain speed of revolution, it tends to keep spinning for some time. When we've built an oscillating pattern of tension, small, insignificant thoughts that by themselves are *not* tension provoking (e.g., a red traffic light will usually not produce tension, unless you're already tense about something else) tend to add themselves to the rhythm and increase its strength. Before long we may feel the full force of tension and anxiety.

Fortunately, the same self-reinforcing process can occur with pleasant thoughts and experiences and can teach us how we might create a natural state of relaxation. Create a mental picture of the following:

Imagine yourself in a mountain meadow. You're sitting by a small stream watching the water tumble over the pebbles. You're especially enjoying the clear air and the fresh scent of the pine trees. You feel completely comfortable; and as you look up toward the high mountains behind you, your body begins to tingle with a feeling of indescribable joy. For a few moments all your problems and tensions disappear as you continue to gaze at the mountain cliffs. With a sense of awe you are completely absorbed in your feelings. The warm sun is shining on you, and you feel at peace and happy.

The selective awareness state of relaxation

We can create an even more profound state of relaxation by selectively focusing our awareness so as to build a rhythm of relaxing thoughts and sensations. We relax the body slowly and rhythmically, concentrate on the rhythm of the breathing, and focus on relaxing scenes and images. Before long we have created a synchronous rhythm of relaxation that tends to sustain itself. Any new thoughts then tend to automatically add themselves to the oscillation. Any thoughts of a tension-producing variety are allowed to pass by unheeded; we give them no energy or we may actually erase them from the conscious mind.

In the state of relaxation thus developed, suggestions can be made to the nonconscious mind that it may then act on. These suggestions will fall into the pattern and become synchronous with the already established rhythm of relaxation. This is what commonly occurs when a patient uses hypnoanesthesia for surgery. Suggestions are given to the patient to numb an arm or leg so surgery can be performed without pain. The suggestions are added into the rhythm of relaxation and accepted by the mind uncritically.

SUZIE

Suzie is a seven-year-old girl who was brought in for emergency treatment of a laceration of her left upper eyelid. Sutures were needed to close the wound, and the area around the eye needed to be anesthetized for this process. Suzie was frightened and crying, and she wasn't about to make it easy for anyone to approach her with a needle. In addition, it was important that she remain absolutely still for the delicate procedure necessary to prevent permanent scarring. The usual way to handle such a situation would have been to hospitalize Suzie for twenty-four hours and use a general anesthetic. Instead we decided to use "natural" anesthesia.

Children are especially good at relaxing and using their imagination. Suzie's case demonstrates all the factors that aid in allowing for the successful use of suggestion. First I asked her, "Would you rather do this the easy way or the hard way?" "The easy way!" she answered. This served as a motivation to encourage her to participate. She was then asked to close her eyes and imagine her favorite television program. Researchers and advertisers have learned that television tends to create a very suggestible state in the watcher. For Suzie, imagining a favorite television show was a good way to focus her attention. Suzie was then led through a series of suggestions to relax her body. The process allowed her to relax deeply and enjoy her internal imagery. The sutures were then placed so as to repair her laceration. She was so absorbed in her imagination and the rhythm of her relaxation that she felt nothing! Minutes later, she returned to her parents, smiling!

There is a great deal of power gained from focusing the attention in a state of relaxation or when the body is functioning in a state of dynamic balance. You have no doubt heard stories of a mother lifting a car off her young child who has been pinned there during an accident. Similar incidents occur during wartime and seem to be the result of focusing the mind selectively on one single task. There are tremendous natural powers in the body that can be put to beneficial use.

There are many ways of creating this rhythmic pattern of relaxation in the mind. Each individual will have his or her own favorite images. Thus the process of relaxation by selective awareness does not lead to any rigidly definable "state." There is no *absolute* level of relaxation. We can only discuss *relative* relaxation. You know your own comfortable state when you call yourself "relaxed." You know whether you are "more" or "less" relaxed than yesterday. Being able to relax and focus attention is the first step in allowing the natural healing processes to work.

The critical factor

Do you ever notice the little voice in the back of your head that always comments on your behavior? Suppose you're at a party and you are a little nervous about meeting some of the people there. As you have a conversation with a new acquaintance, you feel awkward and clumsy. The little voice inside starts: "That was awful; you sounded really stupid. You really sounded naive. He/she probably noticed your trembling and stuttering, etc., etc., etc. . . . "

In a state of relaxation this little voice quiets down, and you are free from the nagging demands, judgments, and criticisms. Close your eyes for a minute and notice how many thoughts pass through your mind. . . . Do the thoughts dart through quickly like the hare in the fable? Is your mind racing? Do some thoughts catch attention more than others? Or do the thoughts pass through slowly like a gently moving stream? Are you aware of the little voice talking to you?—"This is silly." "What's this exercise supposed to prove?" "I'm not doing this right." Or is your critical voice quiet? How relaxed and calm do you feel at this moment?

Relaxation is all too often interrupted by certain kinds of thinking—analytical or *critical* thinking. We can return to the concept of balance to understand this. Critical thinking certainly has its adaptive value; it is necessary at times of danger, in making decisions and plans, in systematic learning, and in countless other ways. You use this mode of thinking to plan time schedules, make sure you get to work on time and fulfill your obligations, to evaluate facts, pay bills, remove yourself from uncomfortable situations, and so on. However, if you begin thinking critically or analytically while painting a picture, relaxing in the sunshine, watching a litter of puppies at play, or while making love, you may find that the joy and enthusiasm disappear. At certain times critical thinking becomes *maladaptive*, and you may find yourself in a state of imbalance where anxiety begins to build.

Imagine an evening with friends where you find yourself laughing, enjoying a wonderful meal, and completely relaxing in a comfortable, familiar environment. Contrast it with an evening where you're constantly aware of time, aware that you probably should be home working, or that you should be careful of the rich food because it might cause you indigestion or weight gain. This evening would certainly be less enjoyable than the first. You can easily see how a pleasant reverie or a joyful occasion can be abruptly halted when your critical factor enters.

The critical factor becomes a stumbling block in learning how to relax. You must remove it before you can relax in the same way you remove it when hearing a joke, reading a story, or watching a movie. It's helpful to begin to notice how much you judge, compare, question, evaluate, analyze, and criticize. Imagine yourself typing a paper quickly and without errors, or producing a beautiful tone on a musical instrument, or gracefully skiing down a mountain. If you now begin to analyze how you're making each movement or try to figure it out, you will begin to make errors and lose some enjoyment at the same time. Try signing your name very slowly, then at the normal speed. The bank cashier will accept only the second signature, the nonconscious one!

Analyzing is a process that requires constant attention and work by the conscious mind. Often we attempt to analyze behavior that is being carried by the nonconscious. When we attempt to break down such a complex behavior as skiing (while we are skiing!), the conscious mind becomes overloaded with details, just as yours did during the exercise a few pages back. The automatic integrated functioning of the nonconscious mind involves far too many components working in synchrony for the conscious mind to analyze in an instant. More and more energy is taken away from the performance of the coordinated activity and put to the hopeless task of consciously breaking it into components. As the connections between the components are broken, the flow and rhythm is interrupted and we take a tumble. The frustration and tension we feel as we sit in the snow is a natural result of our giving our brain an impossible task and our realizing we've "blown it" again. The alternative is to remove the critical factor when it is not adaptive.

Children can teach us how to relax and enjoy ourselves. They seem to have only a fine line between external reality and their internal imagination. They haven't as yet learned analytical thinking and are free to experience the joy of living in the here and now, unburdened by past events or future problems. If we can recall some of that playful freedom and sensitivity, we can begin to *control* the use of our "critical factor" and learn when it's *not* adaptive—in other words, begin to become critical of your use of the critical factor.

Natural relaxation is better than drugs

The awareness that relaxation is important to the healing process is not new. Medical science shows us that relaxation can be produced in many ways. For example, there are drugs that quiet the nervous system, muscle relaxants and pain relievers that interrupt the pain-spasm cycle, and surgery that interrupts the nerve tracts.

Natural relaxation is produced by a change in the way we think and feel—by a change in our awareness of how maladaptive tension puts us into a state of imbalance. It's important to emphasize that we are talking about a process of relaxation that *you* create for yourself, rather than being the passive recipient of drugs or a surgical procedure. Moreover, by rearranging reflexes and nonconscious mechanisms that are maladaptive (rather than by imposing relaxation from the outside through chemical or physical means), the relief may be made permanent and the problem cured.

As you learn to relax yourself, you gain a great deal of power that can be used for maintaining your own health.

Besides eliminating the painful symptoms produced by tension in the body, you can also enjoy the satisfaction of feeling independent and responsible for your own well-being. If you are motivated to do so, you can produce the state of relaxation efficiently so that your natural healing abilities keep your body balanced.

This point of view differs significantly from that held by many practitioners of medicine in our culture, where for many patients there is an almost complete feeling of dependence on the doctor. More and more people are beginning to see how they can rid themselves of lifelong physical and emotional ailments by becoming active participants in their own healing (rebalancing) processes.

3

Emotions and disease

The ass eating thistles

It was harvest time and the master and the reapers were out in the field. When the sun was high in the sky the maidservants loaded the ass with good things to eat and drink and sent him to the field. On his way he noticed a fine large thistle growing in the lane, and being hungry he began to eat it. As he chewed it slowly, he reflected: "How many greedy people would think themselves happy amidst such a variety of delicacies as I am carrying. But for my taste, this bitter, prickly thistle is more savory and appetizing than the most sumptuous banquet."

APPLICATION: One man's meat may be another man's poison.

We all have a distinct, unique, physical appearance. Our emotional nature is just as personal. Each of us has our own unique temperament. You have probably had the

31

experience of commenting to a friend that he or she appeared sad, only to hear, "I'm not sad, I'm just thoughtful." Calling something an apple or an orange usually leaves little question as to what we're referring to. With emotions, however, words are simply reference points, and often ambiguous ones. We each have an individual way of experiencing and expressing our emotions.

Imagine yourself at home one evening feeling happy and energetic. A good friend whom you haven't seen in several months drops by. Your plans for this evening were just cancelled, and you hadn't really decided what you would do instead. You are delighted to see this old acquaintance, and you have a wonderful evening together . . . .

Now imagine the same circumstances in a different emotional state—you're home one evening feeling a little tired and fatigued. You know you have to hurry through dinner because you've made plans for later in the evening. Your old friend comes to the door, and you feel a little awkward. You feel as though you should be glad to see him or her, but you don't have time to talk now—you're in a hurry—and you're feeling a little frustrated and irritated because your friend just dropped in without calling.

None of us can doubt the extent to which emotions affect our lives. Emotions can completely change the way in which we view a situation. Our emotional reactions often present a more accurate picture of us than do the words we say, even though emotions are among the most complex of behaviors and often can completely mystify us. You have probably said to yourself at one time or another, "I never would have said that if I hadn't been so upset."

Emotional stress and psychological attitude affect our physical health. During times of high emotional tension, a personal crisis, or a change in life style, we often develop physical symptoms. During these times we may also observe that minor physical ailments such as tense shoulders or a nervous stomach become more noticeable. A person with epilepsy, for example, has seizures due to a small area of damage in the brain. Yet this is only a part of the story, for a person may go for years without a seizure and then have several after a series of events leaves him in an anxious emotional state.

Our unique patterns cause us to respond differently to different stimuli or circumstances. Some of us need only a few pleasurable stimuli before feeling really "happy"; others need several nearly perfect days in a row before they trade their frown for a smile. A failure at work or the sudden illness of someone close might cause depression in some of us; we might be out of sorts for days and not acting with our usual efficiency. Others might only feel bad for a few minutes and then begin working harder than ever to "get our minds off the problem." After a day of work and stress, one of us might have a headache; another, a sore neck and shoulders; another, indigestion; still another might become short-tempered and irritable.

Emotional response depends on the present situation, past experiences, and how we anticipate the future. Imagine that you go to buy a new car. The salesman reminds you of a friend you knew years ago but have forgotten. While you talk with the salesman you also think about your old friend, and you begin to remember your life years ago—your old house, your job, the old school—pleasant memories you haven't recalled in years. You feel sentimental and happy. Then you notice a song on the radio—the same song you heard yesterday when the cashier at the grocery store gave you incorrect change and you felt angry. You might feel your muscles tense as you recall the incident. As you continue your conversation about the new car, the salesman asks you about your work, and you suddenly feel nervous and apprehensive as you remember the important promotion interview you have tomorrow. You might notice your heart beating quickly, and your palms become sweaty.

The mind and body are not unchanging chunks of flesh that we carry from place to place. Physical and emotional changes such as these are going on all the time, *whether or not we are aware of them.* Most people, in fact, pay little attention to this ever-present information—thus setting the stage for the development of disease.

Your emotional response in any situation is affected by many factors, both conscious and nonconscious. An attempt to analyze the "causes" of your emotions would lead to a hopeless maze of confusion. The important point here is simply to become aware of the complexity and intricacies of emotions and how emotional and physical responses are inextricably tied together. Have you ever purchased something simply because the salesperson was nice or reminded you of someone you liked?

Imagine two patients with the same disease who are given identical medication. One heals quickly. The other shows no change; he is given an increase in medication and soon begins to develop unpleasant side effects. Now imagine two patients who have just undergone abdominal surgery of the same nature. In one case, the incision heals quickly and painlessly and leaves only a small scar. The second patient develops an infection in his incision and is hospitalized for an additional month, experiencing much pain and discomfort. Why do some skiers heal fractured legs in a few weeks, whereas others with identical injuries take six months? Tetracycline or penicillin may be the drugs of choice for a certain infection, yet some patients get well while others who have apparently the same degree of damage fail to respond.

The resolution of a physical sympton or a disease involves more than a clinical diagnosis of the problem. Each of us responds to drugs, medication, surgery, pain, hospitalization, boredom, discouragement, frustration, injury, and so forth in a unique way.

When physical symptoms begin to occur we may experience fear, anxiety, depression, or anger—none of us likes to be sick. Often these emotions produce an ever-tightening spiral in which we become trapped and more and more out of balance. Emotions can create physical tension that may prevent resolution of a problem. We may feel as if we are being controlled, that we are the victims of unfair circumstances ("Why me?"). A simple alteration in our response can change the entire outcome. Simple—but few of us have ever been taught to consider that we can change our emotional responses, few attempt to do it, and still fewer are successful. It's no wonder that we find ourselves in the same uncomfortable situations, repeating the same patterns over and over, even after we've promised ourselves, "I won't let this happen again!"

FRED

Fred is unhappy with a difficult assignment at work; he's becoming noticeably touchy and anxious. Before long he finds himself arguing with a coworker. He develops a headache, and since he's falling behind in his work, today he rushes through lunch. Later in the afternoon he develops indigestion, and his mood becomes even more sour. When he comes home in the evening, he finds his three-year-old daughter's lollipop stuck on the corner of the chair. Fred is so irritable by this time that he becomes angry at her and at his wife for "goofing off" all day, allowing his child to "run amuck through the house" while he's hard at work. He complains bitterly about his headache and heartburn, which are becoming worse, and takes some aspirin and antacids to hide the symptoms from himself.

Fred will probably have difficult assignments in the future and will probably go through similar emotional upsets and physical symptoms, each time somewhat stronger and less under his control. He has planted the seeds for disease, and if he continues at the same pace without looking at the imbalances in his life, he may find himself with a serious physical ailment.

It becomes more and more difficult to break the cycle each time it occurs—a minor physical symptom creates tension and anxiety, which may worsen the original symptom or cause additional symptoms to appear. In other words, we may make a headache or indigestion *worse* by responding to it with tension and anxiety! If Fred could learn how to relax at the first signs of a headache and pay attention to what his body is telling him, he could prevent the acceleration of this cycle.

4
Tension, anxiety, and physical symptoms

The country mouse and the town mouse

Once upon a time a country mouse who had a friend in town invited him, for old acquaintance's sake, to pay him a visit in the country. Though plain and rough and somewhat frugal in his nature, the country mouse opened his heart and store in honor of an old friend. There was not a carefully stored-up morsel that he did not produce from his larder—peas and barley, cheese parings and nuts—to please the palate of his city-bred guest.

The town mouse, however, turned up his long nose at the rough country fare. "How is it, my friend," he exclaimed, "that you can endure the boredom of living like a toad in a hole? You can't really prefer these solitary rocks and woods to the excitement of the city. You are wasting your time out here in the wilderness. A mouse, you know, does not live forever, one must make the most of life while it lasts. So come with me and I'll show you life and the town."

In the end, the country mouse allowed himself to be persuaded, and the two friends set out together on their journey to town. It was late in the evening when they crept stealthily into the city, and midnight before they reached the great house where the town mouse lived.

On the table of the splendid banquet room were the remains of a lavish feast. It was now the turn of the city mouse to play host. He ran to and fro to supply all the guest's wants. He pressed dish upon dish and dainty upon dainty upon him as though he were waiting on a king. The country mouse, for his part, pretended to feel quite at home, and blessed the good fortune that had wrought such a change in his way of life.

But in the midst of his employment, just as he was beginning to feel contempt for his frugal life in the country, the sound of barking and growling could be heard outside the door.

"What is that?" said the country mouse.

"Oh, that is only the master's dogs," replied the town mouse.

"Only!" replied the visitor in dismay. "I can't say that I like music with my dinner."

At that moment the door flew open and a party of revelers, together with two huge dogs, burst into the room. The affrighted friends jumped from the table and concealed themselves in a far corner of the chamber. At length, when things seemed quiet, the country mouse stole out from his hiding place, and bidding his friend good-bye, whispered in his ear: "This fine way of living may do for those who like it. But give me my barley bread in peace and in security in preference to your dainty fare partaken with fear and trembling."

APPLICATION: A crust eaten in peace is better than a banquet partaken in anxiety.

We will now take a closer look at tension and anxiety. As we have indicated, tension and anxiety are integral parts of most of the diseases we face in our culture. Anxiety refers to an emotion we feel when we are out of balance. It may appear as a feeling of frustration, nervousness, apprehension, worry, fear, or even panic. You may experience anxiety in a variety of circumstances—when you miss a plane, when you are depressed, when you feel overburdened with responsibilities, when you're angry, when something is "hanging over your head," and so on. It may occur when you dwell on a mistake you have made or an unfortunate event in your life.

Anxiety becomes maladaptive if you carry it with you into other parts of your life. Imagine the common situation of a man or woman who comes home from work tired and restless and begins to argue with his or her mate. In fact, the argument or the anger may have nothing whatsoever to do with the situation at home but rather is the result of tensions and anxieties at work that are unexpressed. Have you ever found yourself "taking it out" on your husband, wife, or close friend?

Since tension is believed by physicians to be implicated in so many of the problems and diseases we encounter, it's easy to see why chemical tranquilizers, muscle relaxants, and analgesics (to interrupt the pain-spasm cycle) are the most frequently prescribed medications.

The terms *tension* and *anxiety* are often used interchangeably, since we seldom find one without the other. If you are suddenly awakened in the night by a muscle spasm, you would most likely experience anxiety related to the physical pain. Likewise, if you are anxious about an important meeting, the muscles in your body would reflect the anxiety by beginning to tense up. Instruments such as "lie detectors" demonstrate that the stress of even a "little white lie" produces a tensing of many organ systems.

Tension and anxiety are so common in our culture that we may begin to believe that they are part of our "normal" state. A day of feeling relaxed and free of tension may be a rare pleasure (e.g., "I haven't felt this good in months!"). When tension becomes maladaptive, physical symptoms may begin to appear. Putting up with maladaptive tension or ignoring it seldom helps the problem, and before long we become insensitive to the natural rhythms of our bodies—we forget what it's like to *feel good*! How can this happen?

> Make a fist with your right hand. Now hold it for two minutes. You will feel some tension and strain at first, but before the two minutes are up you'll notice that the tension begins to attenuate; you become less aware of the strain in your hand. Your hand may even become a bit numb!

When muscles of the body are tense often, or for long periods of time, the tense muscles may begin to feel almost "normal" as the sensation declines and sensitivity is lost. As a result (contrary to what you might first expect), when first learning to relax the body and quiet the mind, there may be a period of time during which the body feels *more* uncomfortable. This first stage is a positive sign; sensitivity to internal body processes is renewed, and control over the body can now be established. It has been said that before he can strive to be free, a man must discover that he is a slave. So, too, in order to relax, the body must first feel its tension. Slowly, the body begins to respond to this information. It rebalances itself and the tensions fade away.

How can you become sensitive to your natural body rhythm and keep yourself in a state of balance?

SALLY

Sally is an engineer who was asked to work on a special project for her company that would require extra hours of her time for several weeks. It was a difficult job, but Sally was pleased that she was chosen for the project.

For the first few days of working ten hours a day, she came home exhausted and could barely crawl into bed. After a week she began to feel better; her body adjusted to the stressful pace, and she no longer felt fatigued after a day of work. Sally's body was making an *adaptive* response to the situation, allowing her to be flexible and still remain in balance. Sally continued this pace for another three weeks with few problems. She felt excited and challenged by her work.

Unfortunately, Sally's staff and equipment were inadequate to the amount of work she had to do. After a while, she began to notice that she was beginning to feel more and more unhappy, that her senses were becoming a little dull, that she was beginning to get regular headaches, and that she wasn't enjoying her usual hobbies. This was a cue to Sally that she had stretched her limits for several weeks and that now it was time to take a rest. Her feelings and physical symptoms were the first signs of imbalance.

Sally decided to take a couple of days off. Even though she was on a tight time schedule and under a great deal of pressure, she realized that she needed to give herself a short break; she knew that after a short rest, her work would be more efficient and she would feel much better about it. She realized that she was taking a preventative measure against more serious problems.

Sally had the good sense to listen to the cues from her body; she allowed her natural healing tendencies to put her body back into a state of balance by taking a couple of days off.

In our culture, we often find ourselves ignoring these cues. Have you ever continued to push yourself until you needed a doctor's prescription—muscle relaxants, tranquilizers, and sleeping pills—and then wondered why every day seemed like the "same old grind"? There are many good excuses for not taking care of ourselves—pressure from our employer, the desire to be productive, money, not wanting to get behind, and the like. Many people are beginning to ask themselves the question, "Is it worth the price of my health in the long run?" More and more people are beginning to answer, "No!"

Organ language

It is interesting that without realizing it, we often express the relationship between our emotional stresses and physical symptoms in everyday language. If you mentioned to a fellow worker that your job was "a real headache" or a "pain in the neck," he or she would surely know what you meant. Similarly, the man whose anxiety is keeping him from expressing his thoughts often describes himself as having a "lump in his throat"; or the woman who disagrees with a coworker might find herself saying, "I can't swallow that." You may tell the constant complainer to stop "bellyaching" or a nagging boss who is overburdening you with responsibilities to "get off my back." Have you ever told someone how you really felt and felt relieved to "get it off your chest"? Have you ever had "cold feet," felt "weak in the knees," or been "itching" to do something? We see how easy it is to observe tension and anxiety in everday life.

Muscles, muscles, muscles

One way that maladaptive tension can create problems is through the muscles of the body. There are many different types of muscles—the giant muscles of the thighs and the minute muscles in the walls of the blood vessels; the soft muscle of the intestine and the tough, fibrous muscles of the arms; the rhythmic, smooth muscle of the heart and the powerful muscles of the jaw. The basic function of all muscles is *movement*—the alternate contraction and relaxation that allows the body to function. You can observe this movement in the tightening of the jaw muscles when you crack a nut; in the smooth, peristaltic contractions of the stomach when it is digesting food; and in the bulging of the biceps muscle when you flex your arm. This alternate contraction and expansion is necessary for the normal, healthy functioning of all muscles.

Sometimes muscle contraction is not so smooth and controlled. Abnormal contractions often appear as "knots," "charley horses," or as backaches, indigestion, and headaches. This type of *contraction* is called *muscle spasm*. Spasm differs from normal contraction in that the muscle contracted in spasm tends to remain contracted, and the usual relaxation phase fails to occur. Spasm may be painful as in the case of a headache, or it may take other forms

such as diarrhea or asthma. It is difficult to find an area of
the body where muscles are not present. Thus, nearly
every part of the body is susceptible to tension, spasm,
pain, inflammation, and disease.

In many cases, spasm is an adaptive response of the
body and causes problems only when it gets out of control.
Spasm is a way for the injured muscle to protect itself from
further damage and allow time for repair. The pain or
discomfort of muscle spasm is a signal from the body that
the muscle has been overstressed and needs a rest. Sometimes, for a variety of reasons, the muscle doesn't heal and
remains in spasm. The spasm causes more pain, and the
pain continues to increase the spasm. This mechanism is
called the *pain-spasm cycle*, and it lies at the heart of a sub-
stantial number of our physical symptoms.

Unfortunately, in our culture we often carry a level of
unwanted muscle tension with us most of the time. You
can check this for yourself. Using your fingers, carefully
feel the muscles of your shoulders and neck, especially the
muscles in the back of your neck. If you press firmly, you
may be able to detect tiny areas that are quite tender. You
may even be able to feel the tension and spasm like little
knots or nodules. If you press more firmly on these areas,
you may acutally start to experience the beginning of a
headache. Any time that you are worried or under a great
deal of pressure, you may notice that the tenderness becomes more marked and the spasm easier to feel. Imagine
what it would feel like to rid yourself of the tension in your
neck and shoulders!

We'll look at some common examples of how this
mechanism of muscle spasm can create problems
throughout the body. We'll see how relaxation can be used
to break the pain-spasm cycle and to treat the symptoms in

addition to or in place of usual medical treatments—tranquilizers and pain relievers. As we have mentioned, natural relaxation has the added benefit of giving you the control of your health and well-being. People who have used these processes report not only a relief of painful symptoms but also a tremendous amount of satisfaction for having accomplished it themselves without the usual dependence on drugs.[1]

Headaches

Headaches are one of the most familiar examples of muscle spasm. Medicine has a long list of names for different headaches, including such familiar ones as the "tension headache" and the "migraine." You are probably familiar with the dull, nagging headache; with the headache accompanied by sharp, shooting pains through the head and neck; and with the "splitting headache." The usual remedies include aspirin and pain relievers.

Jan

Jan came in complaining of a splitting headache and spasm in the back of her neck. The headache had persisted for several days. She went through a spasm relief procedure as follows:

Jan spent a few minutes lying down, relaxing her entire body and imagining that her mind was free from tension

---

[1] See the Appendix. The "Applications of Autosuggestion Tape (#10)" Tension Relief section, presents a self-applied technique for this purpose.

and stress. She then began to focus on her headache. The first step was to tighten the muscles in her hand by clenching her fist. She held her fist clenched until she had created tension in her hand equal to that which she felt in her head. She experienced fatigue in her hand and a slight sensation of pain and discomfort. Jan then imagined that her clenched fist was superimposed onto the muscles in her neck that were causing the headache. At this point Jan slowly began to relax her hand. She felt a tingling sensation as the blood began to rush through her fingers.

The tension and spasm generated in her hand were produced *voluntarily* under her control. By creating a spasm voluntarily and then relaxing it, Jan taught her mind how to relieve tension. Since her clenched fist was superimposed onto the muscles that were creating her headache, these muscles *automatically* relaxed when she relaxed her hand. Within several minutes her headache was gone, the muscles in her neck were relaxed, and she had learned a valuable method for relieving tension in her body.

The tension-relaxation exercise is a very basic one that demonstrates how, in a state of relaxation where attention can be acutely focused, ordinarily nonconscious processes can be brought under conscious control.

Asthma

One of the most common problems resulting from muscle spasm is asthma. Contrary to what you might expect, the main problem is *not* that the person is unable to inhale sufficient quantities of air, which is the feeling the asthmatic experiences; rather, there is *too much air* in the lungs, and it is not fully exhaled. The small muscles in the lungs—those surrounding the smallest bronchioles—are contracted, constricting the exit of air. This often occurs because of emotional factors or allergy-causing substances in the bloodstream or in the air. This tightening of the muscles prevents the air from fully escaping out the neck of the little air sacs, the alveoli. Since the asthmatic is not getting fresh air, he attempts to inhale more deeply. This air becomes trapped, and the cycle continues. Further gasps for air yield less and less relief. The wheezes in the chest of a person with such a "bronchospasm" are produced through the same mechanism by which a squeaking sound is produced by stretching the neck of a balloon while the air escapes.

The admission ledgers of hospitals across the country show patient after patient brought in for the treatment of asthma. They are often given emergency injections of drugs or are hospitalized for periods of up to several weeks, during which time some even require intravenous medications. Various forms of physical therapy are also used to alleviate asthma and its complications. Complications from asthma, unpleasant and sometimes dangerous side effects from the drugs used to treat asthma, and even death due to asthma and its complications sometimes ensue. Even following this unpleasant and expensive treatment in the hospital, asthmatic patients may find themselves tied forever to bronchodilators, pills, restricted diets, special exercises, and chemical inhalers, which many find as addictive as the cigarette habit!

People of all ages have asthma. Many have been able to reduce or eliminate their symptoms, even on their first attempt, through the use of relaxation procedures. Further exploration into the psychological aspects associated with their asthmatic condition often leads to permanent alleviation or improvement. The advantages of relaxation techniques over hospitalization and chemical therapy are obvious. Many people are beginning to discover that *if they choose*, they can rid themselves of many of the uncomfortable symptoms caused by asthma.

An interesting demonstration of this treatment of asthma occurred recently at a San Francisco children's hospital. Several children who had been hospitalized for treatment of their asthmatic attacks were brought before an audience of physicians. In order to demonstrate the presence of asthma, the physician, a hypnotherapist, held his microphone to the chest of each child so that the audience could hear the wheezes. He then asked each of the children if they'd like to make their asthma go away. They answered with an overwhelming "Yes!" The physician relaxed the children by asking them to imagine their favorite television program. When they were comfortable and relaxed, he placed his stethoscope to each child's chest; and one by one, he told them to imagine that they could "let go" of the wheezes. Each child did so readily, and to the amazement of all present, the wheezes were gone! While the children were relaxed, their nonconscious minds easily accepted the suggestion to "let go" of the trapped air.

The physician then asked the children to bring the wheezes back. They all began to protest. He explained that if they could make the wheezes go away once, they could do it again, and moreover, they would have better control. The children brought back the wheezes and again relieved them. This demonstrated that the normally involuntary muscles of the chest can be brought under voluntary control. And the children went home!

The stomach and digestive tract

Abnormal contractions in stomach muscle produce the well-known "nervous stomach" and indigestion. Other spasms of muscles along the digestive tract we closely associate with ulcers, gall bladder disease, problems in the large and small intestine, diarrhea, colitis, constipation, and hemorrhoids. Even the little appendix has a muscular wall. Perhaps even some appendicitis attacks may be triggered by spasm of these muscles. Problems of the stomach and digestive tract are usually treated by prescribing a change in diet, muscle relaxants, and rest for the patient. In more serious cases, surgery may be the only answer. Again, self-applied relaxation procedures can eliminate some of these symptoms.

HAL

Hal came in for treatment of an ulcer. He had been suffering from stomach pains for six months. His treatment consisted of a special diet and muscle relaxants. Surgery had been recommended by his physician.

Other members of Hal's family had suffered from stomach problems, and he had always been told that he would probably have to face them, too. Hal's anxiety was becoming maladaptive, and the fear of having to live a life limited and restrained because of his health was too much to bear. That fear combined with Hal's tendency to constantly worry and drive himself without slowing down was causing his stomach pains to worsen.

Hal began to use the processes of deep relaxation to relieve the pain in his stomach. As he began to calm down, he realized that his *own* tension and anxiety were making his

49

stomach problem worse. When he understood this, he gradually began to slow his pace in his daily life. In several weeks his symptoms had disappeared.

Hal had been caught in the vicious cycle that so many of us may experience when we have a painful symptom: The symptom causes anxiety, which may cause either worsening or delayed healing of the symptom, which causes more anxiety, and so on. Relaxation processes allowed him to cut through the cycle and see how it was maladaptive.

The circulatory system

High blood pressure and heart disease are among the most common causes of death in our culture. They are diseases directly related to spasm of the muscles in the cardiovascular system. Angina pectoris (pain in the chest due to spasm of the blood vessels in the walls of the heart and in the heart muscle itself) is often seen to be the direct result of psychological tension. People with this problem are routinely treated with tranquilizers.

It has become common knowledge that angina pectoris as well as the common "heart attack" is found more often in tense individuals. Doctors, lawyers, business men and women, and others who have a high level of psychological stress in their professions or at home are prime candidates for early development of these problems.

Tom

Tom came in to be treated for tachycardia—a rapid, throbbing heartbeat and an abnormal heart rhythm. After light physical exertion, Tom complained of feeling exhausted. He also felt anxiety and fear when he experienced the rapid pounding of his heart. Treatment in the emergency room consisted of pressure on the carotid artery, pressure applied to the eyelids, and strong doses of tranquilizers.

It had never occurred to Tom that he could possibly control his own heart rhythm. He had resigned himself to the use of tranquilizers and to living with the threat of a serious heart problem.

After observing the success of a friend who used some relaxation processes to treat high blood pressure, Tom decided to try some for himself to see if he might be able to control his abnormal heart rhythm. He first learned how to relax the muscles of his eyelids and a procedure for testing them to make sure they were really relaxed. The next time Tom had an attack, he applied his new tools, and he *felt* his heart rhythm return to normal. Sure enough, when tested at a hospital, Tom's heartbeat had returned to normal. Tom had experienced a sudden flash of insight while he was focusing on relaxing his body during the attack of tachycardia. He realized how important his own attitude was in keeping his body healthy. He had been reawakened to the notion that his body had natural healing tools of its own and he needn't be dependent on drugs. He continued to work on relaxation processes that he could use at home every day and was able to learn to control the rhythm of his heart. His medication became unnecessary as his body began to balance itself.

High blood pressure is another common ailment known to be closely associated with stress. The technical name, *hypertension*, is indeed aptly chosen, since it has been shown repeatedly that the degree of psychological tension a person is experiencing will affect his or her blood pressure. Prolonged tension produces permanent elevation of the blood pressure. The initial treatment for high blood pressure usually consists of a prescription for tranquilizers.

Any time you are feeling afraid, worried, or "under pressure," you are likely to have an elevated blood pressure. Usually, your blood pressure falls rapidly to normal as soon as you leave the situation that is creating these feelings. This rapid fall of blood pressure back to normal is a property of healthy blood vessels that allows them to maintain *adaptive* flexibility. As stressful situations grow more and more frequent and as we grow older, the accumulation of unrelieved tension causes the blood vessels throughout the body to become permanently constricted. This constriction of the blood vessels produces greater and greater resistance to blood flow. Imagine trying to blow out a candle through a soft rubber tube. If you begin to constrict the tube by pinching it, you will find that more and more pressure is required for the same amount of air to reach the candle. In the same way, when blood vessels become more and more constricted, a higher blood pressure is needed to pump the blood through the blood vessels, and more work must be done by the heart. The diseases resulting from hypertension and this stress on the heart are many—strokes, heart attacks, kidney disease, angina pectoris, cerebral hemorrhage, and arteriosclerosis, to name a few. These problems are often treated with tranquilizers to calm the patient and muscle relaxants to open the blood vessels and permit a lowered blood pressure. In most cases, however, this symptomatic treatment does not halt the progression of the disease. The life situation responsible for the tension continues, and despite medication the tension returns, breaking through the bonds artificially imposed by the tranquilizers and requiring stronger doses of medication (with its possible side effects) to lower the blood pressure!

With the help of relaxation processes, many have been able to reduce blood vessel spasm. Moreover, there is the added benefit of striking at the actual *cause* of the disorder. Many people with hypertension have been able to decrease or eliminate medication, avoid progression of the disease, and bring the blood pressure back to normal by altering their reflexes to stress through relaxation.

SAM

Sam had a problem with periodic pounding headaches, sweating, and nervousness. Between these episodes he felt normal, and no problems were noted during his annual physical exam.

After several years, however, the blood vessels in Sam's body became less and less able to relax following tense situations and his doctor diagnosed his condition as hypertension. He was placed on the appropriate medication, and his blood pressure returned to normal but with one major side effect—he became impotent.[2]

As a result, Sam decided to try a new approach. He came in for treatment and described his nervous symptoms. When asked what circumstances had caused his symptoms to appear, Sam answered that he noticed them whenever he had to wait in line—at the supermarket, the bank, and so on. He was experiencing these symptoms in spite of his medication.

It is probable that with continued stress in his life the inter-

[2]Some of the other common side effects of antihypertension drugs are drowsiness, dizziness, nausea, and depression.

nal blood pressure "thermostat" would raise his blood pressure again, leading to worsening hypertension and more medication. To stop the progression of the condition, Sam began to learn the tools of deep relaxation and became more sensitive to the situations in his life that were causing him anxiety. He realized that standing in line was only one type of situation that caused his nervous symptoms. As he began to spend ten minutes three times each day relaxing his body and allowing his anxious thoughts to float away, he gradually started to look at his life from a new point of view. While deeply relaxed, he began to replay—one by one—instances in the past when he had been waiting in line. The difference was that now he imagined himself relaxed as he waited. Gradually the deeper levels of his mind began to realize that being relaxed in line was a real possibility. He soon found that waiting in line, as well as other stresses in his life, no longer caused symptoms of nervousness.

Sam realized that life was much more satisfying when he could relax and enjoy it. Within a period of five weeks, Sam's blood pressure returned to normal, and he no longer needed medication. His nervousness and anxiety began to fade away. His problem with impotence also disappeared once he was off the medication. Here we can see how medication may cause a physical problem to worsen if the side effects create more anxiety and tension and how natural relaxation eliminates this danger.

Common sexual problems

Tension in the pelvic area may account for many types of sexual dysfunction including vaginal spasm, pain during intercourse, and painful menstrual periods. The uterus is simply another muscle and need cause no more discomfort through its contractions during menstruation or even during delivery than the contracting biceps muscle of the arm.

JoAnn

JoAnn had a problem with painful menstrual periods. Each month she was forced to stay home for one or two days because of severe spasm.

We discussed that uterine contractions need be no more painful than the contraction of any other muscle in the body and that pain during menstruation is often related to anxiety and confusion during puberty. Many women never become aware that menstruation is the normal shedding process of surface cells lining the uterus and that the contractions of the uterus simply force this blood out. JoAnn recalled her teen-age years and remembered the fear she felt during her first menstrual period. She had been unprepared and immediately associated tension and anxiety with the sensations she felt from her uterus.

JoAnn learned some relaxation procedures and began to focus on the muscles in the walls of her uterus. She practiced the hand clasp method just described in the section on headaches: She contracted her hand and imagined that her hand was her uterus. She practiced squeezing her hand until the tension was the same as she felt in the uterus, and then she relaxed it. This process taught her that she could voluntarily control the contraction and relaxation of her uterine muscles. During her next menstrual period, she used these tools and experienced no further pain.

Back spasm

The large muscles of the back frequently go into spasm, and many days or even weeks may be necessary for the problem to resolve itself. Many people are especially prone to the development of back problems, and the anxiety and worry resulting from pain and disability can often prolong the discomfort. Whether the spasm is due to psychological tension or actual muscle injury, we can eliminate the "overreaction" to back pain through relaxation. Chronic spasm in the back often produces an imbalance in the vertebral column that may account for a person's back "going out." This complication is often relieved by rest, drugs, heat, traction, or by osteopathic or chiropractic manipulation. Relaxation techniques can be used to break the pain-spasm cycle in this sensitive area, allowing a natural physical balance to be restored and leading to more permanent relief.

MARY

Mary came in for treatment of severe back spasm. She injured it while exercising and was afraid that she would have to remain inactive for months. A year ago she had a similar back problem, and she experienced pain and discomfort for four months. She also felt discouraged and frustrated over not being able to return to her regular schedule. Her back became a central concern in everything she did. When she strained it again this time, she felt anxious and unhappy about the gloomy prospects ahead. Exercising was a large part of her daily routine, and the thought of having to give it up again this year for several months only added to the tension.

In discussing the problem, Mary realized that she never really allowed herself to relax. She always had to be "doing" something. When she received an injury she had the tendency to give it the minimum amount of time to heal and then "test" it. Because of this, she added extra stress and strain to her back, which was not yet completely healed, and soon she would find herself down again. She began to realize that *nature takes time to heal* and that the pain in her back was a cue that she should take it easy. She learned some relaxation processes that allowed her to focus on the back spasm without the tension and anxiety of "wanting it to heal as fast as possible so she could get back to her regular activities." She used relaxation methods two or three times a day, and after one and a half weeks she had no further symptoms! She was excited and amazed at what a difference her own attitude made to her healing process.

5
Mind and body—
it's all one

A physician was asked what it was like being a doctor. He said, "I feel like someone on a river bank who keeps hearing the cries of drowning people calling out for help, so I keep jumping in and rescuing them, but every time while I'm giving artificial respiration, I hear another cry for help, and so it goes, jumping in, pulling to shore, applying artificial respiration, jumping in, all day long—you know, I'm so busy I just don't have time to look upstream to see why they're all falling in."

—with acknowledgements to I. K. Zola, 1970

Background

Most people can readily accept that we could all function a lot better with less tension and more relaxation. But at this point some of you may be saying, "Hold on a minute! I can see that relaxation may relieve a tension headache or low back pain, and I can even believe that ulcers can be affected

58

in this way, but slowing your heart and lowering blood pressure—that's harder to swallow. And what's this about asthma and diabetes? Aren't they 'organic' diseases—diseases that are associated with actual physical damage? So how could they be affected by the mind? And now we read about heart disease, and even cancer. Are you saying that some people may actually influence the course of diseases like *these* through relaxation and imagery?"

The answer to your question is an emphatic YES!

I know, you want proof. That's fair enough. We live in a culture that *demands* scientific evidence to validate our notions, in which hearing the experience of other people is often not enough to convince us. This is a scientific culture: "If it moves, research it. If it doesn't move, research it." So, for those of us who want scientific evidence of the interrelationship between mind and body are in luck—there are masses of it. This chapter will give you glimpses into this field of inquiry.

The basic questions are these: What is the scientific evidence that a person's thoughts, emotions and tension contribute to physical disease? And what is the scientific evidence that relaxation and imagery can help reverse the disease process? The questions can be made more specific, such as: Can the conscious mind really have a direct effect on what are called the involuntary functions of the body, like heart rate, bleeding, and gastric secretion, and on complex processes like hardening of the arteries?

Interest in questions of this kind is not new. The ancient epic of Gilgamesh, written on clay tablets about 2000 BC, notes that sadness "makes the heart sick" and that "in the city man perishes with despair in his heart." When the Greek philosopher Epictetus said, "Man is not bothered by things, but by his opinion of things," he anticipated by almost 2000 years modern scientific knowledge about the role of perceptions, cognitions (thoughts), and emotions in the disease process.

In 1628 the famous physician William Harvey wrote, "Every affliction of the mind that is attended with either pain or pleasure, hope or fear, is the cause of an agitation whose influence extends to the heart." These observations are also in full agreement with modern theories concerning chronic stress and heart disease. And in the last century, the eminent French physician Fere, in his book, *The Pathology of Emotions* (1899), linked emotional factors to disorders of respiration, circulation, menstruation, lactation, and infection, as well as to diabetes, gall bladder pain, and other diseases.

These and other provocative statements arose from extensive observations. It has been pointed out, however, that this is the age of science, and scientists go by certain "rules of evidence" in forming and testing theories. In this system, the most solid support for a theory—or "proof"—comes from rigorous testing of the theory in specially designed experiments. It may as well be stated here and now that rigorous proof of that kind will never be available for theories linking health status to mental and emotional factors. The most fundamental reason is that these aspects of people's personal lives cannot be manipulated like chemicals in laboratory test-tubes: it would simply be unethical. Moreover, on the practical level it would be prohibitively difficult.

In the absence of pure experimental data, support for a theory can come from the accumulation of circumstantial evidence. In the case of the mind/body relationship, this kind of support is building rapidly, and some of that information is presented in this chapter.

Now a statement of the obvious: Most people want to make up their own minds about personal matters, and want to make their decisions based on the best available information. If a method is readily available that appears to have benefited many people and has not been shown to have harmful side effects, many people will choose to try it. Their decision is based on the same principle underlying the American Cancer Society's adjuncts concerning preventive checkups, that *uncertainty should not lead to inactivity.* "If one waits for perfect information one will have to wait forever. . . . it is simply impossible to have perfect information before making decisions, and at each point in time, we must do the best we can with the information available at that time."[1]

And finally in this section, some words about why the relationship between the mind and the body is of literally *vital* importance to us all. Most of us suffer to some extent from the "hurry sickness," preferring the quick fix over introspection and involvement. For one thing, it gives us more time for hurrying! Indeed, it's not too hard to imagine a patient who would agree to having a hole drilled in his head if it was recommended by his physician, but if that physician prescribed classes in dance therapy, the patient would think his doctor was crazy—"he must have a hole in his head!"

We are culturally programmed to expect fast cures for our ills—pills and shots, scalpel and stitches. Moreover, we tend to view symptoms like headaches, sore muscles, indigestion and insomnia as mere mechanical problems that just need a squirt of oil, rather than as signals from within that all is not well with the mind/body complex. But for two reasons, this approach is inadequate.

First, the fact is that individual choices and everyday habits play a significant part in the onset and course of most human ailments. That means that most illnesses are, in principle, preventable. It also means that most sickness that does occur is, to a greater or lesser extent, amenable to improvement through our own actions. This fact is the foundation of a gradual revolution taking place in the health care field. It is no longer appropriate to hand all diseases over to an expert for fixing and abdicate all responsibility: we must be active rather than passive participants in the care of our own health.

The second point is that in matters of health, there are more options available than we have generally been aware of. As a former head of the World Health Organization put it, "there is more to health than the mere absence of disease."

[1]American Cancer Society, 1979.

In other words there are higher goals to which we can aspire than the absence of obvious symptoms. Moreover, there are imbalances in the human system that we take for granted, saying "that's life!" — rather than seeing that we have symptoms of some more subtle dis-ease.

In summary, for the vast majority of people the ultimate responsibility for health lies with the individual him- or herself. The pay-off for assuming this responsibility is that there are undreamed of levels of wellness available to us all.[2] This is why the study of the mind/body relationship is what our culture calls a "hot topic."

Selected Findings

Much of the evidence linking mental, emotional, and physical health status comes originally from the fields of sociology and psychology. For example, Dr. Langer and her colleagues at Yale showed that the post-operative course of surgical patients was improved when they used a stress-reducing strategy of selective attention.[3] In particular, patients who perceived themselves to have some measure of personal control in the situation, and exercised that control, used fewer medications for pain relief and sedation.

Even more remarkable, when mothers of children who were hospitalized for tonsillectomy were given information about what would be taking place during their children's stay and had supportive conversations with nurses, their children were found to cope better with the hospital and surgical experience compared to children whose mothers were not helped in this way. Even the children's post-operative

[2] The first complete development of the wellness concept is due to John Travis, *The Wellness Workbook* (Berkeley: Ten Speed Press, 1981).

[3] E.J. Langer, *et al.*, "Reduction of psychological stress in surgical patients." *Journal of Social Psychology, 11* (1975): 166-65.

blood pressure and temperatures were lower! In other words, the information and support reduced the mothers' stress, and this effect was transmitted to their children.[4]

These examples point to the close inter-relationship between mind and body, and among thoughts, feelings, and health, and there are many more. The very thoughts we entertain are accompanied by changes in the chemistry of the brain and the biochemical and physiological processes of the body. The moods we feel affect the immune system, the body's "Department of Defense," a phenomenon studied in the rapidly expanding field of Psychoneuroimmunology. Our emotions are accompanied by Physiological change: in one experiment, even people who contorted their faces according to instructions, without knowing what particular mood they were mimicking, showed the physiological effects associated with that "facial mood."[5]

Perhaps the best known example of this relationship is found with heart disease,[6] and especially the famous "Type A" personality, defined by Drs. Friedman and Rosenman.[7] These investigators—both cardiologists— observed that people who developed heart disease tended to share certain characteristics. The "coronary prone" individuals have an underlying sense of time urgency and what is called "free-floating hostility": they struggle against time and other people, are irritated by trivial things, are impatient, and often have a short fuse. They also tend to be perfectionist, competitive, assertive, and ambitious, so of course they are strongly reinforced for their behavior by our high-pressure goal-

[4]J.K. Skipper and R.C. Leonard, "Children, stress and hospitalization: a field experiment." *Journal of Health and Social Behavior,* 9 (December 1968):235-287.

[5]P. Ekman, University of California, San Francisco. Reported in *Brain/Mind Bulletin,* August 1985.

[6]A. Steptoe, "Psychological factors in cardiovascular disorders." (London: Academic Press, 1981).

[7] *Type "A" behavior and your heart.* (New York: Fawcett, 1977).

oriented society. Subsequent studies suggest that the free-floating hostility is probably the most significant factor.

"Type B" personalities may also be ambitious, but they appear to be more realistic about their achieving and to experience a drive that seems to confer confidence and security rather than to irritate and infuriate. They are more likely to be happy with their lives and to maintain good health.[8]

Many physiological correlates of the stress reaction have been found, including acute increases in blood pressure, adrenaline, and other "stress hormones," and in blood cholesterol, a major risk factor for heart disease and stroke. For example, accountants were found to have elevated cholesterol levels each April 15, right at the tax deadline.[9]

Another result of the mind/body connection is the onset of illness after a period of personal upheaval. It has been observed that when a lot of disturbing events occur in a relatively short time span, people tend to become ill soon thereafter, and with a variety of ailments.[10] It is particularly interesting that emotional and physiological stress can result from both the "good" and the "bad" events in life: getting hired or fired, getting married or divorced, beginning or ending school, or any event that requires you to *change*, all are potential stressors.

Overall, Holmes and Rahe found the most stressful event to be the death of a spouse. In another study this finding was confirmed, finding that the mortality rate of widowers within a year of bereavement was more than ten times higher than that of comparable men whose wives had not

---

[8] R.H. Rosenman, *et al.*, "Coronary heart disease in the Western Collaborative Group Study: final follow-up experience of 8½ years." *Journal of the American Medical Association, 8* (1975):233.

[9] M. Friedman and V. Carroll, "Changes in the serum cholesterol and blood clotting time in men subjected to cyclic variation of occupational stress. *Circulation 18*, (1958):852-61.

[10] T.H. Holmes and R.H. Rahe, "The social readjustment rating scale." *Journal of Psychosomatic Research, 11* (1967):213-18.

died. On the other hand, the widowers were ten times more likely to survive than to die, showing again that it's not just what happens to you that determines your future, but who you are and how you deal with your life.

So, not everyone "goes under." As ever, it takes two to tango, and later research suggests that people who can adapt, or roll with the punches, are resistant to such effects. Dr. Kobasa at the University of Chicago identified *hardiness* as the protective trait. Hardy people (1) see change as a challenge rather than a threat. They are (2) committed to themselves and their actions, (3) believe they can exercise control over their lives and are vigorous in exercising that control. Thus, what might be called a positive attitude appears to insure against illness.[11]

Other researchers have confirmed a relationship between psychological factors and physical health. Dr. Vaillant at Harvard studied men for four decades and found that good mental health was an important determinant of good health later in life.[12] At Johns Hopkins University, Dr. Thomas and his co-workers conducted a study spanning more than 25 years and found relationships between social/psychological factors and subsequent illnesses, including cancer, heart disease, and suicide.[13]

The actual mechanisms that produce and modify disease susceptibility are the object of much research. "We know of a direct pathway between mind and immunity via anatomical connections that wire the brain directly to organs

[11]S.C. Kobasa, "Stressful life events, personality, and health: an inquiry into hardiness." *Journal of Personality & Social Psychology,* 37 (January 1979):1-11.

[12]G.E. Vaillant, "Natural history of male psychological health: effects of mental health on physical health." *New England Journal of Medicine,* 301 (1979):1249-53.

[13]C.B. Thomas and R.L. Greenstreet, "Psychobiological characteristics in youth as predictors of five disease states: suicide, mental illness, hypertension, coronary heart disease and tumor." *Johns Hopkins Medical Journal,* 132 (1973):16-43.

such as the spleen and the thymus gland. We know, too, that hormonal secretions, produced by emotions and thought patterns, provide a second, blood-borne pathway between mind and body.[14]

Perhaps the most controversial subject in this field is cancer. Neoplasia, the development and growth of cancerous tumors, has been broadly explained this way: *Neoplasia arises in a sea of restless cells.* "Restlessness" can derive from many causes. The second century physician Galen observed that women who were depressed were more likely to develop breast cancer than cheerful women. Suggestive evidence continues to be uncovered today linking various cancers to individual differences such as inability to express emotions and coping styles. Studies have strongly suggested that stress lowers anti-cancer type antibody levels, that bereavement depresses white blood cell function, and that there is a connection between stress and cancer.[15]

As more and more information is gathered it is becoming increasingly apparent that every human affliction comes from a confluence of external and internal factors—the environmental factors that influence us, the genes we're born with, *and* the particular ways we handle it all. Our characteristic styles of thinking and feeling have been shown to be closely related to the incidence and severity of a host of ailments, including hay fever and rhinitis (irritated runny nose), thyroid disease, asthma, ulcerative colitis, tuberculo-

---

[14]J. Borysenko and M. Borysenko. "On psychoneruoimmunology: how the mind influences health and disease . . . and how to make the influence beneficial." *Executive Health, 19* (July 1983):10.

[15]B.H. Fox, "Psychosocial factors in the immune system in human cancer. IN R. Adler (ed), *Psychoneruoimmunology.* (New York: Academic Press, 1981):103-158; J.B. Jemmott, *et al.,* "Academic stress, power motivation, and decrease in salivary secretory immunoglobulin A secretion." *Lancet, 1* (1983):1400-02; R.W. Bartop, *et al.,* "Depressed lymphocyte function after bereavement." *Lancet,1* (1977):8016, 834-6; "Stress and cancer: the state of the art, Part 2." *Psychosomatics, 22:3* (1981):207-20.

sis, high blood pressure, low back pain, mononucleosis, and herpes.[16]

Recent research confirms the experience of Norman Cousins, who claims to have cured himself of a degenerative disease from which he had been given no hope of recovering by the medical establishment, through laughter.[17] It now appears that laughter may indeed produce brain chemicals that are beneficial for healing. In any case, laughter and good humor in the right place never hurt anyone.

Since the human mind and body are linked, and since the relationship is a reciprocal one, these examples strongly suggest that most people can positively influence their own health.

Taking Control

I can hear you now, "Okay, so how we react to stress can cause diseases and make them worse. But what I want to know is this: can the opposite of stress—relaxation—protect me from illness? If I'm already sick, can I alter the course by changing my habitual perceptions of the world? Where's the *proof?*" And what *is* the evidence that the mind can be used to help cure illnesses and achieve wellness?

---

[16]See previous references, and: S. Silverman, *Psychological Aspects of Physical Symptoms.* (New York: Appleton-Century-Crofts, 1968); W.D. Gentry, *et al.,* "Habitual anger-coping styles: 1. Effect on mean blood pressure and risk for essential hypertension." *Psychosomatic Medicine, 144* (1982:195-202; C.P. McCreary. J. Turner, and E. Dawson, "Emotional disturbance and chronic low back pain." *Journal of Chronic Disease, 36* (1980):709-715; A.S. Evans and J.C. Niedermen, "Psychosocial risk factors in the development of infectious mononucleosis." *Psychosomatic Medicine, 41*:445-66; M.E. Guinan, *et al.,* "The course of untreated recurrent genital herpes simplex infection in 27 women." *New England Journal of Medicine, 304* (1981):759-63.

[17]Cousins, Norman, *Anatomy of an Illness as Perceived by the Patient.* (New York, NY: Norton, 1979).

As you would expect, scientists have taken a careful and methodical approach in addressing these questions. This is done by studying the Autonomic Nervous System. The Autonomic Nervous System has also been known as the involuntary system, because it was for many years thought to be "automatic" and beyond voluntary control. But that notion has been revised, since it has been shown that even lower animals can be trained to make dramatic changes in the functions of their autonomic nervous systems.

In one experiment, rats were trained to modify their kidney function, probably through altering blood flow, by rewarding them for urine formation. Experimental rats have also been trained to alter blood flow so that one ear becomes hot while the other remains cool, on the command of the experimenter. They have also been trained to vary blood pressure and heart rate separately, all by the simple technique of repeatedly rewarding the desired change.

Humans can also learn to control usually involuntary processes. Probably the most widely known examples of such control comes from the yogic practices developed over thousands of years in the Indian sub-continent—men who can survive taking only one breath every fifteen minutes, lower and raise the temperature of their bodies at will, and lower their heart rates to extremely low levels. In recent years many practitioners have been examined in western laboratories and their abilities confirmed.

Rather than spend years in the disciplines of yoga, human beings can learn the techniques of such control with the aid of "biofeedback." With this method, functions of which people are ordinarily unaware, like heart rate and skin temperature, are "fed back," generally with the use of a light or buzzer as indicator. By relaxing and experimenting with various mental images most people can learn to change the internal feeling state so as to cause the indicator to respond, and with practice can learn to modify the bodily function causing the response. The techniques you are learning in this book are the ones most commonly used in biofeedback therapy, and with regular practice you can achieve the same results even without the electronic device. As you learn to relax, you become more sensitive to your inner signals — thus achieving a kind of internal biofeedback loop.

Human volunteers have learned to modify and maintain their heart rates at randomly selected values within an accuracy of ninety milliseconds. The biofeedback machine used to train them looked like an arcade game where the object is to drive a little car so it stays on the road by turning the wheel. These people learned to adjust their imagery and internal state so as to "drive" their hearts between two vertical lines — and the only reward they had was the enjoyment of playing the game!

With biofeedback technology, human subjects have been taught to change the size of their pupils, alter the flow of stomach acid, fire a single brain cell or neuromuscular unit, vary the electrical resistance of the skin, and change the testicular production of sperm. The techniques of biofeedback have been used clinically in the treatment of a variety of conditions, including stroke, high blood pressure, gastric problems, impaired hand function, cardiovascular disorders, Raynaud's disease, shoulder subluxation, and insomnia.[18]

Lowering High Blood Pressure

High blood pressure, sometimes called hypertension, is a condition that affects about half the adult American population. It is a major contributor to heart disease, the leading cause of death in this country. What's more, in 90 per cent of these cases, no specific cause can be found for the increase in the resistance of the blood vessels which is responsible for the pressure elevation. As you can imagine, the idea of lowering blood pressure by relaxation and imagery is an attractive

[18]J.M. Ferguson and C. Barr Taylor (eds), *The Comprehensive Handbook of Behavioral Medicine, Volume 1: Systems Intervention.* (New York: Spectrum Publications, 1980).

one, especially since the drugs employed to do the job usually have unpleasant side effects.

Chandra H. Patel—a cardiologist working in Britain— used yogic relaxation methods assisted by biofeedback (with "GSR," or galvanic skin response) in twenty hypertensive patients. Five of the twenty experienced such great improvement from daily exercises of deep relaxation and imagery that antihypertensive medications were no longer needed. Seven other patients were able to cut back on their dosage by about 50 percent.[19]

In subsequent work, this group of researchers gave health education and training in various stress management techniques to a group of people at increased risk for heart disease. Four years later, there was a significantly lower incidence of high blood pressure, cardiovascular symptoms, and death than would have been expected without the intervention.[20]

Dozens of other studies have reported favorable results in lowering blood pressure and reducing coronary risk using various approaches to relaxation and imagery, including autogenic training, hypnosis, meditation, and yoga.[21]

The positive effects of relaxation methods have also

[19] C.H. Patel, "Yoga and biofeedback in the management of hypertension." *Lancet, ii* (1973):10535.

[20] C. Patel, *et al.*, "Trial of relaxation in reducing coronary risk: four year follow up." *British Medical Journal, 290* (April 13, 1985):11036.

[21] e.g. H. Benson, *et al.*, "Decreased blood pressure in borderline hypertensive subjects who practiced meditation. *Journal of Chronic Disease, 27* (1974):16396; K.K. Datey, *et al.*, "'Shavasan': a yogic exercise in the management of hypertension." *Angiology, 20* (1969):325-33; W. Luthe, *Autogenic Therapy, Volumes I – VI.* (New York: Grune & Stratton, 1969); N. Muskal, *et al.*, "The effect of meditation training on aspects of coronary-prone behavior." *Perceptual & Motor Skills, 58* (1984):515-18.

been reported in the treatment of migraine,[22] epilepsy,[23] as well as pain control.[24]

Relaxation therapy has also been used to reduce the nausea that usually follows cancer chemotherapy, for example, at the Sloan Kettering Cancer Center in New York, where guided imagery is used.[25] Other workers have made use of the same principles in attempts to influence the progression of cancer,[26] and simply to help cancer patients adapt to their condition. There is work being done on the potential of hypnosis that has implications for extension to self-hypnosis in the treatment of cancer.[27]

Certainly the area of cancer is a sensitive one, and therapeutic claims are inevitably and rightly controversial. But some facts seem clear, and they carry an undeniable message of hope. First, the results of studies such as those of Dr. Thomas at Johns Hopkins University (cited in the previous section) show that certain personality traits, habitual coping styles, and psychological factors are related to the

[22] J.D. Sargent, E.E. Green, E.D. Walters, "Preliminary report on the use of autogenic feedback techniques in the treatment of migraines and tension headaches." *Psychosomatic Medicine, 35* (1973):129-35.

[23] M.B. Sterman, "Neurophysiological and clinical studies of sensorimotor, E.E.G., biofeedback training: some effects on epilepsy" IN L. Birk, (ed), *Seminars in Psychiatry,* 5:4,507-25,1074.

[24] e.g. S.N. Haynes, D. Mosely, and W.T. McGowan, "Relaxation training and biofeedback in the reduction of frontalis muscle tension." *Psychophysiology, 12* (1975):547-42.

[25] Reported IN *International Medical World News* (June 1985).

[26] O.C. Simonton, S. Matthews-Simonton, and J. Creighton. *Getting Well Again: A Step-by-Step Self-Help Guide to Overcoming Cancer for Patients and their Families.* (Los Angeles: Tarcher, 1978).

[27] H. Long, S. Longo, and R. Dixon, "The effect of hypnosis on T and B cell function. Paper presented at the 33rd annual workshop and scientific meeting. *Society for Clinical and Experimental Hypnosis,* Portland, Oregon (1981).

subsequent development of cancer. Second, we know that attitudinal factors affect the processes that are involved in the formation and growth of cancer. And we also know that habitual reactions of thoughts and feelings *can* be modified. It is important to leave all elements of judgment outside of this arena where they belong. There is no fault or blame in illness, and no one has to feel guilt for becoming or remaining ill. What *is* worthy of our attention is an honest, realistic appraisal of our respective responsibilities and capabilities.

Many clinicians are now using relaxation and imagery with cancer patients with the twofold aim of improving attitude through self-image change and mobilizing the person's self-healing potential. Patients learn to visualize armies of white blood cells attacking and destroying the tumor, and they are strongly exhorted to picture themselves as recovering from their disease and as being well. We will return to this approach in detail in Chapter 11.

A General View of Disease Susceptibility

Let's summarize what these research findings seem to indicate. The development of a disease in an individual is dependent on many factors. Besides the obvious contribution of genetics and environmental factors like bacteria and toxic chemicals, it is clear that there are at least two other very important contributions: the individual's personality and self image; and the number, severity, frequency and recency of life stresses. Thus we are seeing that many of the factors that combine to produce disease are potentially within our personal control. Moreover, there are psychophysiological techniques available that allow us to alter the course of many diseases, and, better still, prevent them.

Now It's Your Turn

Central to most of these techniques is the process of deep relaxation and self-imagery. The following suggestions will help you get started in using these skills for improving your life and creating your own good health.

Practical Suggestions for Personal Change

1. Go gradually, one problem at a time. Trying to lose forty pounds, learn Chinese, develop a stress management program and make a career change all at once is asking a lot of yourself; take it easy.

2. Define the problem. Write it down very specifically, then list the "pros and cons" of the behavior you want to change (remember that tension, anxiety and physical symptoms are behaviors just as much as cigarette smoking and overeating is)—the benefits you derive from it and the secondary problems it brings. Be honest with yourself, write down everything you think of, and spend some time reading what you've written. For example: "I get headaches at work in the afternoon. My headaches stop me from working so hard, they give me something to be angry about, they give me an excuse to avoid social and work related obligations. They are uncomfortable, they diminish the quality of my work, they last into evening and prevent me from enjoying an active social life."

3. Define your goal, and write it down in detail. Make it simple, measurable and attainable: "By the end of six weeks, I will be free of headaches, I will be more assertive and exercising regularly." Imagine how you will be when it's achieved.

4. Keep records. A diary is a powerful aid to change. Make columns for What, When, How Often, Where, How Much, and Comments. You can record calories, minutes, pulse rates, miles, thought, feelings— anything that's important to you. Set aside a few minutes each day to do this. Every now and then, check yourself out and see how you're progressing. If you haven't done what you wanted or expected, can you see why not? If you repeatedly fail to reach a particular goal, perhaps the timing is wrong, so revise your goal to one you know you can achieve. THIS IS *YOUR* PROGRAM.

5. Counteract negative mental chatter with positive thoughts. If you keep thinking, "Oh, I'll never make it, it's too hard," silently repeat to yourself something like, "I've done difficult things before and I can do this one too." Counteract "I am just the anxious type," with "If I use deep relaxation and imagery regularly, I'll let go of anxiety and feel confident.

Remember—You're doing this for you. You are worth the effort. As long as you're trying, you're not a failure. If you feel your motivation slipping, enlist support from family and friends.

Preparing to Relax

1. Be comfortable. Let your whole body sink downwards, imagining it being attracted by the force of gravity.
2. If you lie down, let you spine sink towards the surface you are on, especially at the waist level. When lying on a flat surface, it usually helps to raise your knees, with your feet about shoulder width apart and the toes pointing inwards *just a little* to keep your knees from falling outwards.
3. If you are in a reclining position, let your spine sink into the chair. If you sit upright, keep your spine vertical so you don't put any strain on your back muscles, but stay relaxed, keep your chin tucked gently in, your neck gently long, and don't try to hold your shoulders up.
4. Breathe from your diaphragm, so that your lower belly, or abdomen, rises a little as you breathe in, and sinks back as you exhale. Imagine a balloon inflating and deflating in your belly. Don't hold in your belly, military style—let it "hang out."
5. Relaxation and imagery are best done in a room that has soft, gentle lighting. A shaded lamp is better than a ceiling light, and both are better than a fluorescent lamp.
6. Arrange your practice session so that you won't be interrupted by the telephone, family, or visitors (you can put a note on the door, leave the phone off the hook).
7. Practice in a quiet place. If there are disturbing sounds, it's often better to "white them out" with a steady background noise like a fan or an air conditioner. Best of all, use stereo earphones—the ear-cap kinds are the best.
8. Keeping your eyes closed can help you concentrate. You may need to open them a few times at first to follow the instructions, but eventually you'll probably want to close them. You can take your glasses off too.

9. You may become more relaxed than you're used to, and even feel that you're out of control—*you're not*. Just clench a fist, open your eyes, voice a sound, and you'll soon see who's in charge!
10. Don't worry if you find you have a stream of thoughts going through your mind while you're practicing— that's true for most people. Let the thoughts come and go, without paying them any particular attention. If you find your mind following a train of thought, don't get upset—just let the thought go and focus back on the instructions.
11. Don't tell yourself you're doing this wrong. There's no one "right way" of doing it. Exactly what you're doing is right for you at the time—this is absolutely true. Like all skills, this one takes learning and practice. You'll become more expert with time.

Basic Relaxation and Self-Imagery Exercise

1. Allowing yourself to rest in your relaxed position, choose some object in the distance to look at and keep your eyes fixed upon it and repeat silently to yourself "There's no place I have to go right now, nothing I have to do and no problem I have to solve . . . I give myself permission to relax."
2. After repeating these words several times and really hearing their meaning, let your eyelids close and take a deep breath in, filling your abdomen, your middle chest and your upper chest. Hold this breath for a moment without closing off your throat, then let it go, imagining that as you breathe out, you're breathing all unnecessary tension out of your body. As you breathe out repeat to yourself the words, "Letting go . . . and relaxing." Repeat two times.
3. Now let the air breathe you, thinking to yourself with each breath in, "It breathes me."
4. Bring your awareness to your feet, and with each breath out imagine all tension is draining out of your feet, like sand flowing out of an hour glass.
5. After about 15-30 seconds, move your awareness to your legs and knees and thighs, and with each breath out, imagine all tension is draining from them. Continue this for 15-30 seconds.
6. Continue through your body in this manner, relaxing your pelvis, your abdomen, lower back, your chest and upper back, your hands and arms, your shoulders and neck, your

scalp and face. When you first start, it may take 15 minutes to complete this portion of the exercise, and, if so, you can skip to Step No. 9. Soon, however, you will find that this phase can be carried out in 5 minutes or less and you are ready to go onto mental imagery.

7. You may find that as your body relaxes you become more aware of the unnecessary thoughts that are constantly going through your mind. Imagine that your nostrils are like two little exhaust pipes that go up into your mind and that with each breath out you are breathing out unnecessary thoughts. Imagine that with each breath in, fresh clean air is being breathed in through your nostrils and is cleansing your mind of unnecessary thoughts. About 30 seconds of relaxing your thoughts in this manner should help you to relax even more deeply.

8. Picture in your mind a very pleasant scene, a place that you would like to go on vacation, perhaps the place you would choose if you could go any place in the whole world you wanted. Bring the scene in clearly and vividly, see the colors, hear the sounds, feel the movement, the physical sensations, smell the smells — really put yourself in this scene.

   Imagine in this scene that you are healthy and well and full of energy. Spend about 2-5 minutes enjoying this place, continuing to breathe unnecessary thoughts out through your nostrils as they come along.

9. Repeat to yourself any affirmations or self-statements that you would like your deeper mind to accept, e.g. "I choose to be healthy. Everyday and every way I'm getting better and better," etc. Gradually reorient yourself to your physical surroundings as though you are really coming from a deep sleep. Come back slowly, bring with you the relaxation that you enjoyed in your special place. As you open your eyes, repeat to yourself the words, "I am awake, alert, refreshed and clear."

10. Some people become so relaxed it is important that they stand up very slowly and avoid activity such as driving for a few minutes until they feel fully wide- awake again. Most people will find that the relaxation they have created stays with them for awhile. At first this may be only an hour or so, but by practicing on a regular basis, you will find that you can relax yourself more rapidly, and that the results of this relaxation lasts for several hours to a day.

6
Symptomatic treatment of disease

The idiot, the wise man, and the jug

An idiot may be the name given to the ordinary man who consistently misinterprets what happens to him, what he does, or what is brought about by others. He does this so completely plausibly that—for himself and his peers—large areas of life and thought seem logical and true even when they are not.

An idiot of this kind was sent one day with a pitcher to a wise man, to collect some wine.

On the way the idiot, through his own heedlessness—smashed the jar against a rock.

When he arrived at the house of the wise man, he presented him the handle of the pitcher and said:

"So-and-so sent you this pitcher, but a horrid stone stole it from me."

Amused and wishing to test his coherence, the wise man

77

asked: "Since the pitcher is stolen, why do you offer me the handle?"

"I am not such a fool as people say," the idiot told him, "and therefore I have brought the handle to prove my story."

Infectious diseases such as malaria, tuberculosis, smallpox, and polio have been conquered and no longer threaten us. We can attribute this success to modern medical science and its advanced technology. Modern medicine has developed excellent surgical procedures—it is possible to relieve obstructions to blood flow within the heart, to remove diseased parts of the body, and even to replace major organs to restore the health of the patient. We have accumulated vast amounts of knowledge about serums, antibiotics, vaccines, and organ transplants; and with purified fluids, we can sustain life through intravenous feedings. The array of equipment used in hospitals staggers the imagination—laser beams, surgical devices for operating on the retina of the eye, artificial kidney machines for extracting poisons from the blood, and heart–lung bypass machines, that allow direct operation on these vital organs while their function is assumed by the machines, to name a few. Yet there is more.

The other side of the coin is that such devices do not enable us to treat many of the problems we suffer from in our culture. There is a definitive treatment procedure for only a minority of diseases. The standard medical treatment for most diseases and physical ailments is *symptomatic*. We treat headaches with pain relievers and analgesics, infections with antibiotics, muscle spasms with relaxants and tranquilizers, and heart disease with vasodilators. Since we are treating only the symptoms, the underlying causes and the conditions that produce them are often left untouched. In many cases, these underlying causes are likely to create similar symptoms or more serious ones in the future. As I've mentioned, at least 90 percent of all of the physical problems and diseases with which we're most familiar have a component of tension. If we treat only the symptoms of disease, ignoring the fact that stress and tension may play a large part in the underlying cause, we may be doing ourselves more harm than good!

The pain that accompanies physical symptoms is a sign of imbalance in the body. If we remove the pain (our cue that an imbalance exists) and are no longer aware of the imbalance, we run the risk of its continuing unnoticed and becoming much more serious. Symptoms are important signs and may indicate that we need to consider the conditions that led to them. Our goal with the processes we've been discussing is to relieve the symptoms *and* explore the cause of the symptoms so that it does not return in the future either in the same or in a different form.

Sometimes symptoms seem to be the body's way of forcing us to take a much needed rest. The overworked businessperson can gain several weeks of rest if he or she begins to develop an ulcerlike pain or hypertension, although he or she would never have dreamed of slowing down otherwise. The actress with a stressful schedule who develops painful headaches around bright lights is forced to take a rest. A sudden cold may necessitate several days of rest for the fatigued student. Symptoms occur when we have ignored imbalances too long. Imagine how much more enjoyable life would be if we could learn to listen to our body cues that tell us it's time for a break, *before* the physical symptoms appear!

Surprising as it may seem, teaching patients to control the underlying processes of health problems does *not* form a part of standard medical treatment. Generally, when we go to a doctor, he or she makes a diagnosis on the basis of our signs and symptoms and our medical history. Personal communication and recognition of the lifestyle and environment of the patient usually play a small, often nonexistent, part of treatment. In medical school, the psychological components of health problems are certainly mentioned, but no methods are taught to deal practically with them.

Far too many people use the admitted shortcomings of the medical and surgical field as an excuse to avoid seeing physicians for symptoms that we don't understand. Sitting in a doctor's office waiting to hear a diagnosis from a doctor who has to look on your chart to even remember your name is often far from a pleasant experience. Many people have a fear of physicians dating from a painful experience with hospitals and doctors. Such childhood, phobiclike reactions can be dangerous. Often a disease that is curable in its early stages may develop to the point where it becomes debilitating, and complications result.

The person with a pain in the abdomen may suspect an ulcer. He or she may imagine that a doctor will order rest at home for several weeks. This may be such an unpleasant thought that he or she may delay going until the pain becomes much more severe and there is no choice. How different it might be if the individual could go to a physician and be taught some relaxation processes whereby to learn to reduce stress and cope better with his or her job and decrease the tension associated with the abdominal pain.

Learning to reduce the tension underlying physical

symptoms by no means makes the normal medical diagnosis and treatment unnecessary. An ulcer may be eliminated in its early stages with the aid of relaxation processes; but once it has formed a hole in the wall of the stomach and hydrochloric acid is flowing into the abdominal cavity, surgery is necessary. Knowing how to relieve the pain of recurrent headaches doesn't negate the necessity of having a doctor determine whether or not they are due to abnormal blood vessels or a brain tumor. Untreated, the underlying process could lead to far worse problems. Combining relaxation procedures with the usual treatment can lead to much more comprehensive and complete medical care and gives the patient some tools to control the stress and imbalance in life.

The proper use of medication

Medication prescribed by a physician can be viewed as an *aid* to the natural healing process of the body. Antibiotics provide an excellent example of how such aids are used. The body is constantly controlling microorganisms such as bacteria, fungi, and viruses so as to keep the body safe from such foreign invaders. The skin, for example, has elaborate defenses to prevent the entrance of organisms that can cause disease. Any organism that passes the skin barrier is quickly attacked by antibodies and white blood cells. Infection often results from an imbalance in the mechanisms that prevent the entrance and reproduction of bacteria. The body attempts to isolate the area of infection, blood flow is increased, and antibodies and white blood cells are rushed to the site of infection. Medication may be prescribed to aid the body in restoring its natural function. Antibiotics don't *heal* the body; they merely weaken and slow the growth of foreign organisms so the body's own defenses and tissue repair mechanisms may gain the upper hand. When this occurs, medication is no longer needed.

The fact that antibiotics work as *aids* to the healing process is obvious from the following example: Some people suffer from a rare disease involving defects in their white blood cell- or antibody-producing systems. Their health is seriously endangered by even the slightest infection no matter how many antibiotics are taken. Even a boil on the skin can be fatal. In our culture, many of us have been taught to deemphasize the importance of the natural healing process in favor of external medications. It is becoming more and more clear that this priority should be reversed.

In prescribing medication, it is important not to hide the symptoms of a more fundamental process. Just as attempting to eliminate the headache of high blood pressure by covering up its symptoms with codeine can produce serious or even fatal consequences, so, too, can an emotional problem worsen if the symptoms are hidden by tranquilizers. The young man or woman who has chronic acne may be done a disservice if he or she is placed on antibiotics for the infection but never allowed to see that basic feelings of embarrassment and insecurity allow the problem to persist. Continuous suppression of a vaginal infection with medication may keep a woman from examining an unsatisfactory sexual relationship that might be causing the symptoms to appear. The businessman who uses analgesics and tranquilizers to relieve the headache resulting from chronic tension at the office may never examine his job and his relationship to it, continuing to create more tension and stress, which may lead to more serious physical symptoms. Restoring "health" means more than eliminating pain. It also means making sure the body processes are functioning to maintain balance and—equally important in our new definition of *health*—that the individual is also experiencing satisfaction and fulfillment in life.

II
The roots of disease

The ant and the grasshopper

*One frosty autumn day an ant was busily storing away some of the
kernels of wheat which he had gathered during the summer to tide
him over the coming winter.*

*A grasshopper, half perishing from hunger, came limping by.
Perceiving what the industrious ant was doing, he asked for a
morsel from the ant's store to save his life.*

*"What were you doing all during the summer while I was
busy harvesting?" inquired the ant.*

*"Oh," replied the grasshopper, "I was not idle. I was singing
and chirping all day long."*

*"Well," said the ant, smiling grimly as he locked his granary
door, "since you sang all summer, it looks as though you will
have to dance all winter."*

APPLICATION: It is thrifty to prepare today for the wants of
tomorrow.

Introduction to part II

In Part I we saw how relaxation can help to eliminate physical symptoms that are present and prevent new symptoms from occurring by restoring the natural balance of the body. In Part II we explore the roots of disease and how treatment can eliminate the disease patterns completely.

In Chapter 7 we discuss imagination and how it becomes more vivid and creative in a state of relaxation. It is through the imagination that thoughts bubble up from the nonconscious mind and bring new insights to disease symptoms and maladaptive patterns. In this chapter you'll be able to see how central the image you have of yourself is to determining your everyday behavior and how you might adjust it to suit your needs better.

Chapter 8 discusses our evolutionary background and gives you some insight into why maladaptive patterns seem to persist and are so difficult to overcome. In Chapter 9 we explore memory and how the mind stores information and experience. You'll see how the mind uses this information to determine your patterns and your personal characteristics. We can potentially reach back into the past and recover any memory stored in the nonconscious mind. We take a look at the actual process, the *exploration,* by which we trace the roots of symptoms and maladaptive patterns in Chapter 10.

Chapter 11 includes numerous cases of people who have eliminated their maladaptive symptoms and habit patterns. The cases are not presented for you to compare them with your own patterns but rather to give you a picture of how people have transformed their attitudes about health and healing. These changes in attitude have allowed these people to experience dramatic improvements in their health as well as an overall rise in the quality of their lives.

What patterns or habits in your life would you like to be free of? Do any of these patterns seem to persist no matter what you do to overcome them? What physical symptoms do you notice when you become tense and anxious? Think back into your past. . . . What events in your life might have made those areas sensitive? Keep the answers to these questions in mind as you read the cases in Chapter 11; it will help you to clarify your own attitudes on health and healing.

7

Imagination

The magic word

The Three Wisest Men of the Land of Fools, by some lucky chance, met Khidr, walking the Earth trying to impart wisdom.

"Would you like to know the Word whereby everything can be accomplished?" he asked them.

"Yes, indeed," said the Three Wise Men.

Khidr said:

"Are you ready to hear it?"

"Yes, indeed," said they.

So Khidr told them the Word.

The First Wise Man said:

"But this is a word which anyone could pronounce—this cannot be of any use." So he promptly forgot it.

The Second Wise Man said:

"This word is too inelegant for me," and he found that he could not remember it.

The Third Wise Man said:
"It can be written—so it cannot be of any use. It does not sound like what I expected—so it is not the right kind of Magic Word."

Then they all noticed that a deputation of ordinary citizens of the Land of Fools was waiting to hear some of their wisdom, so they hurried off to fulfill their obligations.

To be *imaginative* is a potential of every human being. We all use imagination before carrying out any conscious acitivity. It is the act of forming a mental image of something not necessarily present to the senses. Take a moment to imagine an apple . . . .

Whether you think of a red apple, a sliced apple, a large shiny apple, an apple with a bite out of it, or any number of other possibilities, you are using your unique imagination. To use the imagination to its fullest, it is not necessary to *think* but rather to allow the mind to be receptive; the thoughts will come spontaneously. We all do this all the time automatically, although we may not be aware of doing it. Recall the last time you sat and listened to someone talk and were bored; do you remember how your mind wandered off, following its spontaneous thoughts?

People experience their imagination in different ways. Some tend to "see" images; others "sense" or "feel" them. Nearly everyone has auditory images—voices of friends or parents or the sounds of musical tunes commonly occur. Think of a tune you like. Can you play it in your mind? There are no incorrect ways to experience imagination. To wonder if you are using it correctly is to bring in your critical factor; and as with relaxation, the critical factor brings the imaginative processes to a halt.

Each of us has a vivid, creative imagination. Many of us, however, have forgotten that we have this amazing creative aspect and may have kept it hidden away for years. As we have discussed, our culture rewards us for rational, linear thinking such as is necessary in science, technology, and business. We may often find that our imagination and intuition are criticized, invalidated, and judged as "unscientific"—that "imagination is for children." Our culture has tended to move away from individual or collective human values in favor of production. Human values became submerged in the Industrial Revolution where sameness and standardization became the priorities. Creative imagination and individuality seemed to run against this newly established cultural norm. As children, most of us were taught that imagination and storytelling were only "fantasy" and that organized, rational, objective thought was "real." We are now seeing that the new, emerging frontier in medicine and psychology in our culture is supporting freedom of imagination and creativity. We are beginning to understand how health of the body is linked to the mind and its creative aspects. By viewing the mind and the body as one whole, functioning unit, we can experience more of the rich potentials of being human.

Imagination involves a mechanism by which we record and use information from the environment. When you see something, you then think about it, form a mental picture of it, and add it to your memory; then by using your imagination, you can respond to the mental image as if it were the *real* thing. We can use a vivid movie to demonstrate how powerful this process is. After the movie, you may think about it, form a mental picture of some scene that you vividly recall, and then, by imagining the scene, respond with feelings of the same intensity as when you saw it in the theatre. You may experience fear, anxiety, excitement, sadness, or any other emotions and their physical correlates—increased heartbeat and breathing, sweaty palms, and so on. This may happen even if you're only describing the film to a friend. Even though you *know* it is only a motion picture, your body and mind respond with powerfully strong emotions. We can use this example of how we react to movies to demonstrate how naturally we use imagination all the time.

Imagine yourself sitting in a movie theatre—an enclosed room with an air conditioner and several hundred people around you. Some people are eating popcorn and other snacks, some are chatting, some are walking up and down the aisles. You are sitting comfortably in one of the chairs with your eyes fixed on a plastic screen, yet you completely forget that you are in a theatre as you find yourself absorbed in the movie! You have suspended your critical factor and allowed your imagination to take over. In fact, you may become "lost" in your imagination. You may be happy at one moment, sad the next; and you might lose track of time and your surroundings altogether.

Creative imagination

In a natural state of relaxation, the imagination becomes much more vivid and spontaneous. Thoughts come that we ordinarily wouldn't notice when our minds are filled with other things. We have observed that the conscious mind has limited storage facilities and becomes easily confused and disorganized if too many thoughts or feelings come in at once. You have no doubt experienced that when you are focused on one thing, you can't think of anything else—your mind is filled. The experience of having so much to do that you can't do anything or don't know where to start is a common one. Only when things are taken one at a time can anything be accomplished. Have you ever forgotten someone's name and found that the harder you tried to remember it, the further the name slipped away? When you give up ("Oh, it will come to me later"), you relieve the pressure, and the name may immediately pop into your conscious awareness.

When the mind is faced with too many pressures, it wants to end the ambiguity by finding a solution. Under pressure, the mind will choose a solution that has worked in the past, even though it may not be completely appropriate to the present situation. In other words, under pressure, the mind tends *not* to choose new, creative solutions.

In a relaxed state, the mind is not threatened by ambiguity. By relaxing we temporarily empty our minds of tensions, frustrations, anxieties, and problems. The mind is more free of stereotyped behavior patterns and can react creatively. Old memories can be recalled that we haven't thought of in years. The solutions to problems come through the imagination; and we may think to ourselves, "It seems so simple; why didn't I think of it earlier?"[1]

Imagine that when you are relaxed, your mind is like a coffee percolator. In the beginning, nothing happens.

---

[1]See the Appendix. The cassette tape "Letting Go of Stress" (#23), presents a method of actively applying relaxation to increase creativity.

Then, slowly, imaginative thoughts begin to percolate. After a while, more and more thoughts begin to bubble up from the nonconscious mind where they are stored. We often call the use of our imagination in a relaxed state a *daydream*. You have probably had the experience of daydreaming about a house you'd like to build, a hobby you'd like to start, a summer vacation, or the person you'd like to develop into. You may daydream about how you'd like to look, new ways you'd like to act, your childhood memories, future successes, and the like. When you are relaxed you may be surprised at how clearly you can remember what you thought were "forgotten" memories. Now let's explore how memories from the past can affect our lives *now*!

The self-image

What is your general self-image? Do you get up in the morning happy to greet the day, or would you rather stay beneath the blankets? Do you smile or laugh often? Are you overburdened with responsibilities? Do you stand up straight and speak confidently, or are you shy and retiring? How do you feel and act around your spouse, mate or friends? Are you satisfied with your work, your physical appearance, your emotional responses, your mental abilities? Are you sure of yourself or do you hesitate? Are you capable of making decisions quickly? Do you make many mistakes? Do you punish yourself for your mistakes or do you accept and grow through them? Are you usually on time, or are you often late? Do you see yourself as a leader or a follower? Is your body strong or weak? Are you too fat? Too thin? Do you like social evenings, or would you rather spend a quiet evening at home?

The image you have of yourself is made up of the sensations, thoughts, feelings, interpretations, and experiences that you have accumulated throughout your life. It has a three-dimensional quality, a depth; and you carry it suspended in your mind at all times—whether you are reading, running, sleeping, or talking with friends.

Advertising clearly demonstrates the central importance of the self-image in everyday life. When trying to sell you a product, an advertiser will create a scene that is relaxing and pleasing, then superimpose the name of the product. The message produced in your mind will be, "If you use this product, your life will get better and you will feel the way you would feel in this scene." The cigarette advertisement doesn't say, "Smoke my brand and you'll feel like this cowboy"; if it did, you'd laugh at the ad. Instead, the message comes through subtly, through suggestion, and by-passes your critical factor. If the ad appears often, you see it over and over again, and your nonconscious mind begins to respond. Advertisements promise changes in self-image such as: "You'll be more beautiful (or handsome)"; "you'll feel better"; "more people will like you"; "you'll be the envy of all your friends"; "your love life will improve"; "you'll have a beautiful smile"; "you'll stay calm and fresh all day"; and so on.

You have no doubt had the experience of knowing when it's time to do a little readjusting of the self-image. You may get feelings or sensations from your body that tell you it's time for a change. By paying attention to these feelings you can often lift yourself out of a slump or a rut. You may find yourself saying, "I need to get out of the house for a couple of days"; "I need a new perspective"; "I'm not myself today"; "I'm beside myself"; "I'm tired of the way I look, I think I'll get a new hat"; and so on. It is important that you pay attention to these signs. You may find that you become discouraged and frustrated, tense and anxious, when you ignore these desires. A small change in lifestyle, your normal routine, or appearance can be just the thing that's needed to restore balance.

Often, when a man shaves off his beard or mustache or a woman changes her hair style, it takes several days to become accustomed to the new look. The nonconscious mind still has an image of the "old you." Looking in the mirror may be quite a shock. On the first day after a change in appearance, everyone seems to notice; and the world is viewed with a slightly different perspective. Can you see how central your self-image is in your life?

Your self-image is who you think you are, and sometimes the negative aspects of the self-image can create a state of imbalance where you may find yourself unable to deal with your environment in an adaptive way. The negative aspects of the self-image—the parts of yourself you don't *feel good* about—often become deeply ingrained early in life. You may grow up thinking that you are unattractive, stupid, unsuccessful; that you always come in second (or last!); that you are perpetually sick, tense, anxious; and so on. The way you think of yourself determines how you act in the world. The man or woman who sees himself or herself as a failure will surely make mistakes, have little self-confidence, and will often feel discouraged and unhappy. In other words, your thoughts and feelings about your successes, failures, joys, and tragedies are consistent with your self-image.

The information coming through the senses from the environment can be blocked, distorted, limited, and misinterpreted by the self-image. Imagine the college professor who is giving a speech to a group of faculty members at her university. She comes home feeling angry and upset—feeling that she has given a poor talk and embarrassed herself in front of her peers. An hour later, a fellow faculty member calls to compliment her on her excellent lecture. Our college professor is surprised, and only after several minutes of praise can she begin to believe her friend. She has an image of herself as being awkward and clumsy around her peers, and her self-image distorts her perceptions so much that she can't believe that a fellow professor could actually have enjoyed her speech.

Imagine a group of young boys who are rock climbing. One of the boys, Tom, doesn't want to go. He complains that he's accident prone and will probably fall. The other boys persuade him to come along. He carefully makes his way along the edges of the rocks, checking his footing at every step and wishing he were as quick and agile as the other boys. Soon he finds himself behind, and while hurrying to catch up he slips and twists he ankle. He yells ahead to the other boys that he will wait for them at the bottom of the ridge and unhappily begins to climb down. In this case, Tom's self-image limits his activities to "safe" sports where he won't get hurt and where he can't feel unhappy and inadequate around his friends. His accident seems to prove the correctness of his self-image.

The self-image can easily misinterpret reality. How often have you been convinced that you did poorly on an exam and then been surprised to find a good grade on your paper? How many times have you met someone who was convinced that he or she was unattractive, stupid, or weak when it was obvious to you and everyone else that the exact opposite was more true? Then there is the person who believes he or she is the best at everything, seemingly unaware that there are few who would agree with this self-assessment!

Changing your self-image can change your life

If so much of your self-image is built when you are young, how can you change it? We all have areas of our self-image that we'd like to be rid of. Changing the self-image is *not* merely positive thinking. We all know of the person who tries over and over again, working as hard as he or she can, and continually fails in spite of good intentions. It doesn't work to *think* positively if we hold a negative self-image! We *can* learn to *accept ourselves* and minimize the misinterpretations and distortions of the self-image; we can learn to "see ourselves the way we really are."

The self-image is highly resistant to change. The heavy smoker who smokes three packs of cigarettes a day, the overweight college student who can't resist a dessert, or the businessperson who continually fails promotion exams all create a state of imbalance with their self-image; they continue to repeat behaviors that have no adaptive value. The smoker doesn't want to smoke but can't help it. The image he or she carries in the mind is one of a chain smoker. The college student doesn't feel good about overeating but can't seem to stop. The image he or she constantly carries is one of being fat and uncomfortable. The businessperson has studied long hours for weeks to pass the exam but is so nervous during the test that it's impossible to think. He or she carries around an image of him-/herself as a failure—he/she sees him-/herself as always working hard but never quite making it to the top. These people don't want to have these maladaptive habits, but they don't know how to change them.

The mind seems to pay special attention to negative aspects of the self-image. You may occasionally find yourself so overwhelmed by one aspect that it may affect your entire outlook on life. Imagine the woman who refuses to go to parties or to go out with friends until she loses a few pounds. Losing weight becomes the most important task in her life, and her perceptions of everything around her become distorted. No matter what she is doing, she is constantly aware of the extra pounds that are keeping her from feeling good about herself. She thinks that her friends won't want to see her, because she has an image of herself being "ugly" when she's a few pounds overweight. Or imagine the small child who has such a great fear of dogs that he won't walk to school with the other neighborhood children and refuses to go outside to play if there are any dogs in sight. His whole relationship to his peer group is affected.

A negative self-image might also cause you to underestimate your own skills and keep you from expanding your talents and expressing your creativity. What you actually can do and what you *think* you can do may be quite different. Imagine the talented young artist who has support and praise from her friends and family for her beautiful paintings but refuses to sell them or show them in an exhibit because her self-image continually tells her that she's "not good enough." Everyone who sees the paintings remarks on their excellent quality, yet the artist cannot see this.

Let's look at an example of how the self-image can cause physical changes in the body.

HAL

Hal is a high school student. For most of his life he has been shy and withdrawn. Most of his friends have girlfriends and Hal feels left out. For the past two years Hal has had a serious acne problem. He's used medication after medication with no success. Hal's thought of himself as ugly for years, and now his skin problems proves to him that he's right!

It was clear that Hal's skin condition had some emotional roots. After talking with Hal about self-image, he decided to try an experiment. Each morning when he got up he would go to the mirror, point to each pimple, and say, "This is exactly where it's supposed to be." Within two weeks there was a noticeable change in Hal's skin condition, and in a few more weeks the acne was completely gone.

By noticing the pimples and accepting them, Hal began to change his self-image. As long as he had an image of himself as being "ugly" he would feel that way, and the tension of the muscles in the skin would prevent the glands from emptying. He realized that he no longer had to hide from his friends; if he could accept his skin problem, so could they. He began to build a realistic picture of himself. Rather then carrying around the idea that he was ugly and that no one would like him because of it, he began to realize that he simply *had acne*. With that acceptance, he no longer needed the pimples to "prove" anything to him, and so they disappeared.

GEORGE

George had just been in a skiing accident and suffered a broken arm. As he was being taken to the hospital, he felt severe pain in his arm and shoulder. His mind began to race with a train of thoughts. "Will I be able to write? . . . Can I stand the pain of having it set? . . . How long will I have to be in the hospital? . . . I'll miss work; how will I pay my bills? . . . How could I have been so stupid! . . . If only I hadn't. . . .

When George arrived at the hospital he was shaking and tense; he was given tranquilizers to calm him. The doctor found it difficult to set his arm because of the spasm in the surrounding muscles. George experienced great discomfort from the cast, and the bones took an especially long time to heal.

Of course anyone who is in an accident will experience some pain, tension, anxiety, and fear of disability. However, by using relaxation and imagination, pain can be minimized, recovery time shortened, and the psychological attitude of the person improves as well. What happens when relaxation and imagination are combined to create a self-image that will allow a quick return to balance and health?

JOE

Joe was scheduled for surgery to have a hip joint replaced. He hadn't been able to walk well for eight months and had been continually out of work. He could have scheduled surgery earlier, but he couldn't bear the thought of such a serious operation and the long recovery period. He had a great deal of fear about his hospitalization and came in to see if he could change his attitude for the better. The pain in his hip was becoming more and more severe, and the tension and anxiety created by the pain were becoming more and more maladaptive.

Through relaxation Joe learned how to control his maladaptive fear responses. In the deeply relaxed state of selective awareness he imagined situations where his legs were strong and flexible. He imagined the night before the surgery—he would sleep well and wake up feeling relaxed and comfortable. He pictured himself being wheeled into the operating room and drifting into a comfortable, deep, relaxed sleep requiring a minimum of anesthesia. He imagined himself after the surgery waking up in the recovery room and the doctor telling him that the surgery had gone remarkably well. He would feel relaxed and hungry (to prevent postoperative nausea), and he imagined himself urinating soon after surgery (to prevent postoperative urinary retention). He imagined himself free of discomfort, needing no pain shots or medication. . . . Joe then used relaxation tools to prepare himself so that he would be able to leave the hospital in record time.

The day of the surgery Joe felt calm. He had been practicing for several weeks. His surgery went smoothly as he had imagined with no complications, and he needed *no* postoperative medication even though the surgeon had totally replaced both hip joints. He surprised the medical staff with his rapid healing. Joe's case is an example that demonstrates the importance of motivation for the success of these processes. He had been willing to face his original fear of surgery and responsibly began to change his self-image so that he would be prepared.

Negative self-images can become the *roots* of physical problems and disease. Deep relaxation and imagination can be combined to adjust the self-image and restore harmony and well-being. As you begin the process of adjusting your self-image to express yourself "as you really are" with less distortion and misinterpretation and begin to see clearly both your faults and your skills, you will no longer be trapped in the maladaptive patterns that make you uncomfortable and unhappy. You will gain a greater appreciation for and acceptance of yourself.[2]

---

[2]See Appendix. The "Applications of Autosuggestion Tape (#10)," is designed to help you create and strengthen your self-image.

8
The nature of man

The crow and the pitcher

A crow, so thirsty that he could not even caw, came upon a pitcher which once had been full of water. But when he put his beak into the pitcher's mouth he found that only a little water was left in it. Strain and strive as he might, he was not able to reach far enough down to get at it. He tried to break the pitcher, then to overturn it, but his strength was not equal to the task.

Just as he was about to give up in despair, a thought came to him. He picked up a pebble and dropped it into the pitcher. Then he took another pebble and dropped that into the pitcher. One by one he kept dropping pebbles into the pitcher until the water mounted to the brim. Then perching himself upon the handle he drank and drank until his thirst was quenched.

APPLICATION: Necessity is the mother of invention.

Once a negative aspect is built into the self-image, it becomes highly resistant to change. We may understand that it is maladaptive, we may make a conscious decision to change, try again and again to eliminate it, and find that it still persists!

We can begin to understand why this is so by looking back at the evolutionary process of Homo sapiens, the human being. The most important point to be aware of is that the human animal, like other animals, is oriented toward survival—to find food, shelter, and safety from danger. Any situation that threatens survival causes an increase in tension in the body so that we can quickly and effectively cope with the danger. The rise in tension and the subsequent readiness for rapid behavioral response is automatic and instinctive—we don't need to learn it.

Imagine one of our *Homo sapiens* ancestors many thousands of years ago living in a cave. He had two kinds of processes that allowed him to survive—exploratory behavior, which allowed him to search for food, shelter, and comfort, and "fight or flight" behavior, which protected him from danger.

Imagine a group of deer browsing in a meadow for food. They are extremely hungry and have traveled a long distance to find the lush meadow, yet the sudden appearance of a predator or an unfamiliar sound will instantly send them running off to find safety. The nervous system undergoes a marked change to prepare an animal for fight or flight. For example, the blood flow to the intestines is halted by contraction of muscles surrounding the intestinal blood vessels, and the blood is shunted to the muscles of the legs. The blood pressure increases to ensure adequate circulation to the brain, tear glands empty to prevent drying of the eyes, and the heart rate and breathing increase. Only after they are certain that danger has passed will the deer relax and cautiously venture back into the meadow.

We are much like the deer in the meadow. The human body undergoes a similar transformation when the mind signals *Danger!* One of the reasons that people are often obsessed with thoughts about the negative and tension-producing aspects of their daily lives is that our minds naturally tend to focus on the situations of highest tension and anxiety, since those are the situations that seem to threaten our survival. Let's look at two examples of how our ancestors probably made use of these characteristics.

In the first instance, we can see how exploratory behavior can replace habitual patterns which are no longer adaptive. In the second example, we will look at a situation where survival is threatened and a high level of tension is created, and we'll see why this response persists in an adaptive way long after the danger passes to protect against future danger.

Suppose the cave man has located water some distance from the entrance to his cave. To reach the water hole, he takes the same winding path through the woods each day. Before long, a change in the weather leads to a drying up of the water hole. That same day the cave man follows his usual path through the forest and finds no water. Surprised and confused, he checks his tracks to make sure he has come to the right spot. He comes back again the next day to see if the condition is the same. By this time, he has realized that he must immediately begin to search for a new source of water and abandons his old habit of going to the water hole. His motivation to find a new source of water comes from the tension in his body created by thirst. We see how easily an old pattern is eliminated when one is motivated by more urgent needs. Can you think of patterns that you have abandoned for similar reasons in your life?

What about other habits? Why do some persist indefinitely? Imagine the cave man when he is a young boy of three or four. While climbing around on the rocks outside his cave, he falls off a ledge and scrapes his knees. Immediately his mind sees steep ledges as a threat to survival and records the situation. He will not fall off many ledges before he gets the message that he must be cautious. Even though he may not be around rocky ledges again for years, he will remember that they are dangerous. When he approaches one, he will feel a rise of tension in his body, reminding him to be alert. He will keep a safe distance from the edge of the rocks. The permanent recording of events that threaten survival is necessary in order that we learn how to protect ourselves. Unlike the vast majority of higher animals, our species lacks strength, speed, agility, endurance, and other well-developed physical defenses. Our one major defense is our sensitive brain and nervous system. With our central nervous system, we can detect danger, develop novel and effective defenses, and protect ourselves.

Twentieth-century "fight or flight"

We can easily see that our *natural* tendency is to respond to dangerous situations—high places, thorny plants, deep water, and predatory animals—because they may be a threat to our survival. On the other hand, these natural responses can cause quite a problem in our present world. In our modern society we fear circumstances that cause us no actual, immediate physical harm. We fear nuclear war, economic collapse, sexual frustration, personal failure, loneliness, cancer, heart attacks, automobile accidents, and pollution. We are afraid of speaking in front of groups of people, of failing in our work, of confronting a friend we are angry with, of talking to strangers, of being rejected by someone we admire, and so on. Though our minds have become highly developed and we no longer live in a primitive environment, our bodies still respond to high levels of tension in the same way our ancestors did. Our muscles tense, our blood pressure and pulse rate go up, and digestion is interrupted when we perceive a threat. We experience anxiety, but the "fight or flight" responses used by our ancestors are no longer appropriate. Whether we are being attacked by an angry lion or by an angry boss, the "cave man" mentality of the nonconscious mind simply interprets that we are being bodily threatened. But if our boss is yelling at us, we can't run away or strike back. Our social structure prevents the natural response, and we find ourselves in a situation the cave man never experienced. We block our natural responses by inhibiting their expression. Our muscles get tighter; we become more anxious. A headache develops . . . perhaps indigestion . . . high blood pressure. . . . Should we ignore the symptoms? They only get worse due to the vicious pain-spasm cycle. When there is an excess of tension in the body, it demands attention. Should we take a tranquilizer or muscle relaxant? The basic problems remain, and the escape through artificial "relief" can make them even more serious. We may need more and more medication. Should we surgically remove the problem area? The anxiety eventually finds another target.

When the body realizes it needs relief from the internal pressure and it looks for an escape, anything that provides relaxation or a temporary release from tension can become a habit—smoking, drinking, overeating. The tensions and anxieties may begin to multiply until we are faced with a debilitating disease. . . . If your employer is angry with you or you feel rejected by someone you love, where can you go to escape?

Hospitals are filled with people who have been unable to find relief from tension—tension produced by stress, physical pain, frustration, anger, discouragement, a persistent maladaptive habit pattern, or maladaptive fears.

Imagine that a friend of yours has claustrophobia and cannot ride in an elevator. He or she chooses to walk ten or twelve flights up a dark stairway rather than take the elevator. Explaining that there is nothing to fear or demonstrating your own confidence in the elevator and its inch-thick cable seldom reduces the tension. The little girl with a fear of snakes is not helped by her brother who holds her while a friend approaches her with a harmless snake to show her that it doesn't bite.

Imagine an overweight man who forces himself to stay away from food. He becomes depressed, anxious, and may have unexplainable surges in temper. Finally something happens that is really upsetting, and diet or not, he opens the refrigerator and pulls out a snack. He feels relieved for a while, since the natural response of the body to food is relaxation—and he has escaped from the tension. Soon, however, he begins to think about how he failed in his efforts to lose weight once again. He becomes tense and angry with himself and soon finds himself eating to relax—and the vicious cycle continues even stronger. And when he goes on another diet, it will be even harder not to eat. Locking the refrigerator door won't change his habit.

Consider the escape drinker. After only the first, second, or third drink of her life she doesn't have a *habit*.
There seems to be no danger; it relaxes her, and she continues to drink alcohol occasionally, especially in tense
situations. Before long, in situations of pressure and stress,
she begins to automatically reach for a drink. Soon she
may start drinking whenever minor tensions arise, and
before she knows it, she may find herself drinking
throughout the day. Alcohol has become a way for her to
escape from her tensions.

A cigarette habit may become established in the same
way. The cigarette that was once a welcome relief from
pressure has become mandatory. Once he is hooked the
smoker finds the habit is a constant source of potential
tension; if he does not have a cigarette he feels internal
pressure. He doesn't want to smoke, but now his reactions
are so automatic that he finds it almost impossible to stop.
He may view his smoking as a major problem if he has
frequent bronchitis or high blood pressure. Though he
may want to stop smoking and is encouraged by his family
and his doctor, he may still be trapped in a repetitive pattern.

Maladaptive habits begin in situations of physical tension and are associated with emotional anxiety. The situation is recorded in detail by the nonconscious mind. The
next time a similar situation or a similar feeling of tension
occurs, the mind feels a threat to survival is present, and it
reproduces all the behaviors that were present in earlier
situations in the hopes that one of them will result in escape; i.e., you tend to attempt to escape from tensions in
the same old ways. The means by which the cave man
learned to avoid rocky ledges now works against us. Thus
if you have a marital problem and drink alcohol for a few

nights as a relief, you will tend to drink heavily during future domestic disputes. Once you begin to act out a familiar pattern of behavior, that pattern will continue to be strengthened with time. After a few times, you begin to react automatically, and you begin to see yourself as responding a certain way—you have created a piece of your self-image.

Many cigarette smokers consume far more cigarettes per hour when working at their desks or while driving in heavy traffic than while relaxing on the beach; still others smoke more when in social situations. Obviously, this is not a simple need for the drug, nicotine; the culprits are tension and faulty self-image.

After a maladaptive pattern has been learned, you soon "forget" the original situation where you first experienced the behavior and years later wonder why your habit is so hard to break. You may struggle, make resolutions and promises to yourself, and still find it difficult to break the cycle. The way to eliminate the problem is to learn to relax and go back to your self-image and adjust it or expand it. Hiding your cigarettes or locking the refrigerator only changes the *external* circumstances and won't work.

9
The earliest memories

The three tradesmen

The enemy stood outside the walls of a certain city. As they brought up their siege weapons and arranged their forces for the attack, the desperate defenders within held a council of war to determine the best means of holding their city.

A bricklayer arose. "Sirs," he said, "it is my opinion that the best material for this purpose is brick." Then he sat down.

A carpenter asked to be recognized. "I beg to differ with the bricklayer. The material that will best serve our desperate needs is wood. Let timber be our defense!"

Then a tanner jumped to his feet. "Citizens," he cried, "when you all have had your say, I wish to remind you that there is nothing in the world like leather!"

APPLICATION: It is difficult to see beyond one's own nose.

112

Evidence has accumulated that indicates that the mind seems to record all the significant events of our lives, including the experience of birth. Generally, as we grow older, these events remain stored in the nonconscious mind and seem forgotten. Yet it is the significant events of our childhood years that lead us to form our self-image—sometimes maladaptively.

Many people have recalled memories from their first years of life while in a deep state of relaxation.

SUE

Sue's experience is a clear demonstration of how the mind recalls and stores events throughout our lives. She came in to explore whether or not it was possible to remember events from her early childhood. She decided that she would try to recall the first day that she walked. Consciously, Sue had no recall of the event. In a deep state of relaxation she began to focus on her childhood memories and specifically on the day she first learned to walk. While she was relaxed and her mind uncluttered with thoughts, Sue could allow old memories to bubble up from the nonconscious. Through her imagination, she began to get images of the living room of the house where she grew up. She described her mother, father, and grandmother in vivid detail, down to the expressions on their faces and the clothes they were wearing. She recalled standing up and slowly walking toward her mother who was sitting on the sofa. She remembered toppling over a few times but also recalled a feeling of great satisfaction that she could now walk on two feet like everyone else in the house. Sue clearly recalled the couch—the shape of its arms, the small tufts of material on it, the color, and the pattern.

After the session, we discussed her experience. Sue was pleased that her memory had been so vivid and alive and was quite convinced that her mind could store the complex details of her past. One point confused her, however. In the state of deep relaxation, she clearly recalled the couch on which her mother was sitting; yet she had no conscious memory of any couch like the one she described. To resolve the confusion, we called her older brother, and Sue described the couch to him. He was amazed that she could remember so well a couch that had been sold before her second birthday to make room for a new one! She had been correct in her description, even down to the little tufts on the cushions.

Through the use of deep relaxation and imagination, we can potentially reach any event in our past. This has powerful implications for finding the roots of disease. Here are some examples of how the mind records experience.

PHIL

Phil is an artist who came in for treatment of back pain. He was also experiencing a growing dissatisfaction and discontentment with his art. In a state of deep relaxation he recalled a memory out of his past:

. . . Phil is three years old and is being taken to the hospital for a tonsillectomy. He is fighting and screaming while the doctor is examining him. Finally, he has to be strapped down so he can't move. As he is squirming and struggling to free himself, the anesthesiologist puts an anesthesia mask over his face. The last thing he remembers before the surgery is the strain in his back from being tied down and twisting to get free. Hours later he wakes up with a sore throat and a feeling that something has been taken away from him. . . .

Phil's case demonstrates the power of the nonconscious mind to recall events of early childhood. It also clearly demonstrates that the brain has a clear image of each of the bodily organs. For years, Phil has been a modern, free-form sculptor. He has created many giant aluminum objects that have a similar style. Though not obvious to Phil, having no background in physiology, the sculptures look remarkably like tonsils! One sculpture shows a vivid rear view of the tonsils, the shape of an artery that makes a loop to go around the Eustachian tube, and the lymphatic adenoid tissue surrounding the area! Only those who study anatomy would know how a pair of tonsils look from this perspective.

It appears that through his art work, Phil's mind was constantly attempting to recapture something he had lost. He realized that the tension in his back began early in his childhood and was related to the anxiety, fear, and feelings of rejection that he had associated to being strapped down before the operation. This is an example of how a traumatic event such as Phil's tonsillectomy can leave permanent impressions on the self-image and therefore affect behavior for years to come.

DOREEN

Doreen came in for treatment of an overweight condition. She continually ate too much and felt ugly as a result. Her depression over the way she looked caused her to eat more, and the cycle continued. In a state of deep relaxation, she heard her mother's words at the moment of her birth: "Oh my God, she's ugly." Doreen's mind had stored every detail of her birth, along with the trauma and the increased tension. At that time, of course, she didn't know what the words meant—she hadn't learned English yet! Even at this early age, her mind began to build an image of being "ugly." Her mother began to breast-feed her shortly after birth, and as a result her first tensions became associated with feeding and feeling hungry. As she grew up, Doreen began to create the circumstances that would fill her self-image. Every time she was anxious or afraid, she would eat. She would then feel ugly, which would trigger anxiety, which would in turn cause her to eat.

Only after recalling the memory in a state of relaxation and selective awareness could Doreen begin to understand the reasons for her mother's remark—her mother's fear, the dulling of her mind with anesthesia, and her unpreparedness for the sight of her child at birth. Once she could see how she had created the image of herself as being "ugly" and that it was not adaptive, she began to readjust and expand it. This allowed her to be in control of her compulsive eating. No longer did tension and anxiety lead her to the refrigerator. And she began to lose weight!

Though her memory seemed real enough to her, Doreen found it hard to believe that her mother, who loved her so dearly, could ever have said such a thing. So she decided to talk to her mother and check it out. In reply, her mother became very upset and exclaimed angrily, "Dr. Roberts must have told you, he's the only one who heard me and he promised never to tell anyone!"

These are dramatic examples of how memories can be recovered from early childhood. In most cases, however, only a small percentage of memories recovered in therapy go back this far. Resolution of a disease, symptom, or maladaptive emotion doesn't always depend on the discovery of a hidden traumatic event of childhood. Often the memories are "familiar"—recalled from the past few years or even from recent weeks. The important factor is an emotional reliving of specific situations (which may or may not have been temporarily forgotten) where a maladaptive behavior pattern is present, then tracing it as far back through time as possible, often to the "very first time the emotion and the pattern ever occurred." In this way, seemingly unrelated events are connected through an emotional linkage; this can then provide a deep insight about the behavior and related emotions, which can then be changed.

You may be surprised that the mind can so clearly store events and words from even the first months of life, though obviously the infant could not possibly understand them. A familiar example might make it more reasonable. Many of us as children learned songs like "Frère Jacques," "Allouette, Gentille Allouette," or "Hava Nagila" long before we had any idea of what the words meant. Perhaps the brain of the infant, alerted by the fight or flight chemicals in the blood stream, simply records the event. Later, when language has been learned, the event is interpreted entirely in the nonconscious part of the mind, and events and words are taken at face value.

Is it hard for you to believe that a child at birth after nine months in the womb is capable of such complicated mental activity? Imagine the child who is born after seven months (premature birth). By the time it is two months old, it has learned to smile, to focus its eyes, and to perform other complicated activity; yet its brain is exactly the same developmentally as that of the newborn of nine months' gestational age, though the full-term baby shows no evidence of having learned anything. Experience shows us that the thinking mechanism is developed long before birth. The last few months in utero seem to be devoted almost entirely to development of muscle and fatty tissue. From these observations and recent evidence that considerable learning goes on during the last few months in the womb, it is not too great a leap to consider the possibility that a preverbal child's brain can record accurate memory traces of words.

Under ordinary conditions, we often resist recalling painful events ("I don't want to talk about it; it just makes me sad"). This is especially true of children. The nonconscious mind tends to "hide" the memories that would cause fear and tension. The event is stored clearly in the nonconscious mind but may eventually become inaccessible to *conscious* awareness. It is doubtful that Doreen would ever have recalled her birth experience consciously just by wondering what the source or her eating habits were. Only a state that would by-pass the critical factor and provide the safety of deep relaxation could allow this painful discovery.

Many of us seek in vain to *figure out* our problems and wonder why they occur over and over again. Rational thinking does not overcome fear. Like the deer in the meadow who sees a mountain lion, we also must *escape*. Merely attempting to recall events and emotions in our normal waking state may fail to help us change a pattern, because of the natural mechanism by which we escape from threatening or fearful situations. The mind will resist recalling a traumatic event. Perhaps you've discussed with a friend an event that occurred years ago. You might remember your friend as being sad and unhappy at the time, whereas he or she has no recollection of those emotions whatsoever. You might have seen a photograph taken on a day that you've since remembered as happy and joyful, only to discover that your expression in the picture is sad. Can you recall hearing a tune on the radio and feeling that you must turn it off because it evokes sad memories? Perhaps you avoid a certain street, a restaurant, or a social environment or group because of certain memories there. Memories associated with tragedy, pain, fear, and even love and joy may overwhelm you with emotion. But such memories can be useful in a state of relaxation, where they are not threatening and can help us trace the roots of disease.

The doctor's repeated warning to the patient that his or her health will improve as soon as smoking is eliminated often doesn't do much good. Rationally explaining to a child with a fear of dogs that dogs are lovable, harmless pets also doesn't help. The nonconscious mind is irrational; therefore, trying to figure things out by controlling behavior with the conscious mind is usually a useless task. What we can do is create an environment of relaxation for ourselves and let the nonconscious mind begin to percolate—to bring up thoughts spontaneously and automatically and *then* look at them rationally to clarify them and see how they've affected our lives. By understanding how these memories affect our self-image, we can also begin to free ourselves from the guilt we often feel when we promise ourselves that we'll change a habit pattern and fail.

10
The exploration

The Tale of the sands

A stream, from its source in far-off mountains, passing through every kind and description of countryside, at last reached the sands of the desert. Just as it had crossed every other barrier, the stream tried to cross this one; but it found that as fast as it ran into the sand, its water disappeared.

It was convinced, however, that its destiny was across this desert; and yet there was no way. Now a hidden voice, coming from the desert itself, whispered: "The wind crosses the desert; and so can the stream."

The stream objected that it was dashing itself against the sand, and only getting absorbed; that the wind could fly, and this was why it could cross a desert.

"By hurtling in your own accustomed way you cannot get across. You will either disappear or become a marsh. You must allow the wind to carry you over, to your destination."

But how could this happen? "By allowing yourself to be absorbed in the wind."

This idea was not acceptable to the stream. After all, it had never been absorbed before. It did not want to lose its individuality. And once having lost it, how was one to know that it could ever be regained?

"The wind," said the sand, "performs this function. It takes up water, carries it over the desert, and then lets it fall again. Falling as rain, the water again becomes a river."

"How can I know that this is true?"

"It is so, and if you do not believe it, you cannot become more than a quagmire; and even that could take many, many years; and it certainly is not the same as a stream."

"You cannot in either case remain so," the whisper said. "Your essential part is carried away and forms a stream again. You are called what you are even today because you do not know which part of you is the essential one."

When he heard this, certain echoes began to arise in the thoughts of the stream. Dimly, he remembered a state in which he–or some part of him, was it?–had been held in the arms of a wind. He also remembered–or did he?–that this was the real thing, not necessarily the obvious thing, to do.

And the stream raised his vapour into the welcoming arms of the wind, which gently and easily bore it upwards and along, letting it fall softly as soon as they reached the roof of a mountain, many, many miles away. And because he had had his doubts, the stream was able to remember and record more strongly in his mind the details of the experience. He reflected, "Yes, now I have learned my true identity."

The stream was learning. But the sands whispered: "We know because we see it happen day after day and because we, the sands, extend from the riverside all the way to the mountains."

And that is why it is said that the way in which the Stream of Life is to continue on its journey is written in the Sands.

None of us is born with smoking problems, an unreasonable fear of snakes, anxieties about speaking in front of a large group of people, allergies, migraine headaches, or high blood pressure. Yet few of us probably remember the exact point in our lives when we first noticed an unwanted physical symptom or a maladaptive habit pattern. Before we realized what had happened, we may have begun to make comments like, "I know I smoke too much, but I just can't seem to quit"; "I know I should slow down and relax, but there's always so much work to do"; "I know I should evercise my body, but I just don't have the time"; or "Whenever I'm under pressure, I get a tension headache." Whether or not we've ever thought about it, then, there was some situation or series of situations in which our bodies, minds, and emotions were trained to respond in this odd manner.

But why should this paragon of evolution, the human brain, record and retain such patterns? One of the major functions of the nervous system is to help us to adapt. It painstakingly learns for us the mechanics of walking, talking, and writing by trial and error, selecting responses that move us in the direction we choose, lead us to pleasure and satisfaction, protect us from pain—in other words, it functions nonstop around the clock to help us adapt. We are thus led to consider that at one time our now troublesome responses were viewed as adaptive.

Very often this is due to the misinterpretation of a situation and the selection of a seemingly appropriate response that later proves to be detrimental. When this response is learned by the nonconscious mind, it becomes as automatic as our signature or style of walking; and it will seem to resist conscious efforts to change it.

Perhaps you've had a conscious experience of misinterpreting an event and responding in a way that would have been different had you known all the facts.

BONNIE

Bonnie was brought to the emergency room after swallowing the contents of a bottle of sleeping pills. She had been experiencing marital problems for several months, and they were getting worse. Last night she had a serious argument with her husband and she was desperate! Her husband stormed out of the house, saying that he couldn't cope with her mood swings any longer. He didn't come back that night, and Bonnie was convinced that he had left for good.

The next morning, while grocery shopping, she saw her husband walking toward his car with his arm around the shoulder of a woman in a green dress. She did not see the woman's face but was convinced that the worst had happened. She became very upset and was brought to the hospital by her family, crying and in a state of panic and despair.

Shortly afterwards, her husband heard the news and came to the hospital; with him was the woman in the green dress. Bonnie sat bolt upright in bed, her eyes big as saucers; the woman was her sister-in-law! Her husband had been so confused and upset by their argument that he had driven that night to a distant town where he spent several hours talking with his sister. She had returned with him, intending to help. When Bonnie saw them at the shopping center, they had just eaten breakfast and were on their way home to see her and try to resolve the problem.

Bonnie burst into tears again, but this time for a different reason. She was happy to find that she had been wrong, and the panic and despair began to disappear. No one could really blame her for her emotional response—she had misunderstood the circumstances. Seeing things in the right perspective completely and dramatically changed her emotional state.

In this example, the maladaptive nature of the emotions was brought to light and the problem was resolved. But what about those situations where strong emotions have resulted from misunderstandings and the nonconscious mind seems to have hidden them from conscious awareness?

Maladaptive patterns can lead to disease and painful physical symptoms. We will begin to focus on the process through which we combine relaxation and imagination to explore the nonconscious memories that may lead to disease and to bring them into the realm of the conscious mind for consideration. The process we use to trace memories back to the source of a physical symptom or disease is called the *exploration*. The situation(s) that causes a high degree of tension or fear to be associated with an organ of the body or with a behavioral response pattern is called the *sensitizing event(s)*. Subsequent similar events strengthen the association.

A sample exploration

Imagine that you are about to undergo an exploration. The first step is for you to define your specific goal—the elimination of a recurrent disease, a physical symptom, a maladaptive emotion or habit pattern. For example, you might wish to find out which situations cause your belly to tighten up and what specific parts of those situations are the triggers that have eventuated in your ulcer or colitis. You might be interested in exploring to determine the early events that have programmed you to feel nervous in front of people that you don't know well. Or you might wish to explore a habit of eating, drinking, or smoking too much—with a goal of discovering what events in your life programmed you into having these automatic responses and what triggers are responsible for maintaining them.

The next step is for you to become as comfortable and relaxed as possible. The selective awareness state of relaxation—a deep meditative state, or a light to medium state of hypnosis—is an excellent point from which to begin. During such relaxation, communication with nonconscious improves considerably. Generally, when I am working with an individual, this relaxation process takes from three to seven minutes and is characterized by feelings of warmth, relaxation, and lightness in the body and a clarity of mind with a relative freedom from intruding thoughts (mind chatter). I help the person enter this state through suggestions of relaxation. I'll describe the exploration just as though you and I were in the same room and I were guiding you through it. An exploration without a guide is quite possible but requires some amount of training.

You are sitting or lying in a comfortable position, quiet and relaxed with your eyes closed; your body is very relaxed, and your mind is relatively free of any pressures or anxiety. Although only the voluntary muscular system can directly relax, as deeper levels of relaxation are reached, relaxation is induced in the internal organs and their involuntary muscles. Further mental relaxation is produced by allowing you to focus for a while on a very relaxing scene such as a favorite vacation spot or a place where you could "get away from it all." Now that you are relaxed and comfortable and your mind is clear, you can begin to allow thoughts to bubble up from the nonconscious mind by allowing it to guide your imagination. Whenever a person stops trying to consciously direct the imagination, the nonconscious will take over and lead it.

Now let yourself drift back to some time in the recent past, a few moments before you experienced the problem that we are exploring. Thus I might suggest that you go back to just one minute before you lost your temper some time recently, one minute before you had the urge to smoke a cigarette, or one minute before there was an event that caused an internal tension that eventually produced a migraine headache. The deeper levels of your mind will choose the memory for you. You may be surprised at the one that occurs to you and for a moment may think that it is not the "correct one"; but remember—the decision is made by the nonconscious part of your mind, which does not follow the same rules of choice as does the conscious part. The nonconscious, however, holds all the memories of your life experiences, and the ones that it chooses for you will fall into a pattern that will give you an insight into the problem you are working on. Since this first memory is a very recent one, it could obviously have been made conscious without the prior relaxation, but in this state you will be more aware of details and of specific emotions that may have gone unnoticed by you in the original experience.

Now, starting from one moment before the critical spot in your memory, we slowly proceed through it, reexperiencing as many aspects of the scene as you can—seeing it, hearing it, and feeling it emotionally to the degree that you can, just as though it were happening—you are more aware of each of your reactions and responses that may have been automatic in the past.

Now that this memory has been completed, clear your mind again by erasing all thoughts, questions, and images. Judgments and attempts to "figure things out" by the mind are distractions that could interfere with the exploration; thus they are erased whenever they occur during the exploration.

Now drift back to an earlier memory just one moment before a very similar pattern occurred. This may be back several weeks or several months. Now relive this scene as vividly as possible, paying attention to every aspect of it. As you reach the point where the pattern is being triggered, you will feel a certain emotion within. Locate this emotion in your body when you feel it—it may be a tightening in your chest or throat or a feeling of wanting to run in your legs. You may notice a sad, angry, frightened, annoyed, hopeless, or other unpleasant emotion as you go through this part of the scene. Amplify this emotion; your ability to recognize it will enable you to change the pattern. After you have experienced this scene as fully as possible, take a deep breath in; and as you let it out, let this scene fade away as you did the previous one.

Gradually, one by one, you recall more and more memories drifting back to earlier and earlier periods in your life. As you enter each memory focus on it and it alone, and make no attempt to relate it to the other memories. This prevents the familiar mental tricks of intellectualization and rationalization from interfering. In each memory, your focus is primarily on the emotions associated with the memories, and often such strong emotions occur that tears result. Let them flow. This is a part of the process of opening yourself to the possibility of a new level of understanding. During the exploration, people often discover hidden relationships between emotions and physical symptoms.

After we have gone through several memories, generally five to ten, I suggest that you go back to the very first time in your life that you experienced this symptom, maladaptive habit, or emotion—the sensitizing event. Actually a true "sensitizing event" occurs only in a minority of instances. Most of the time, there is actually a series of very early experiences in which a painful emotion and a maladaptive reaction occurred together. In response to this suggestion, then, the nonconscious mind would come up with one of those earliest experiences, and this would serve our purposes quite well.

Often this event or series occurred years ago, sometimes back in the very earliest years of life. Once again, this memory is lived with full emotional awareness.

Now let this memory fade from your mind, become completely relaxed again, and return to the present. Now, while remaining relaxed, look at the series of memories that you relived a little while ago. Let yourself see from a much more relaxed point of view what happened in each memory and how you reacted. Let youself see how the memories are connected together in various ways—similar emotions, similar body sensations and physical symptoms, similar habit patterns employed in order to escape from the emotional pressure, similar environments, relationships, and so forth. Often the earliest of these memories prove quite revealing, especially when physical symptoms and a high level of fear are part of the original problem.

The earliest memory of a real estate salesman who felt

nervous and uncomfortable around strangers was an experience of becoming lost in a supermarket at the age of two. Although his mother probably found him within a minute or two, in the mind of a child this young, it seemed an eternity. Subsequent events of being separated from his mother in groups of people merely served to strengthen this basic fear.

An actress with chronic indigestion and abdominal pain reexperienced a memory of when she was three years old, in which her four-year-old brother punched her in the stomach to try to get back a piece of candy of his that she had just eaten.

A man with a long-standing, generalized fear of being trapped went back to a number of experiences in which he was left for long periods in his crib, feeling trapped and helpless.

As you look back from your relaxed perspective, many new aspects of your pattern become clearer to you. Some you may have suspected before, others may be completely new. You now have an insight that can allow you to deprogram the response and provide you with the opportunity to teach your inner mind to be creative in such situations.

Remaining relaxed, you now drift back to the earliest of your experiences. You relive it once again, but this time you change your script. Even though the same events occur, you remain relaxed and confident. You realize that no matter how uncomfortable things might be, relief is not far away and that time will take you to it. You begin to look at creative alternatives for yourself. You choose one of these options and employ it, writing your own script and rewriting this scene.

Now clear this memory from your mind, and turn to

the memory in which you were next oldest. As you look at it from a more adult perspective now, you can make new decisions; and you relive this scene, writing a new script for your body, mind, and emotions.

Step by step we go through each one of these memories, reliving them and rewriting them, always feeling relaxed and confident. Because you felt a good deal of tension the first time through the memories and now feel much relaxation as you go through them, you are demonstrating in a very palatable way to the nonconscious part of your mind that memories it always associated with fear or tension can be viewed in a different manner. In effect, you are desensitizing yourself to the stimuli present within these memories.

You now project ahead to the future situations that contain the same basic elements as those you have reviewed from the past. The difference is that now you have new choices available. If you imagine that your real life extends back into the past along one line like a railroad track and that there is another railroad track consisting of all those memories that you have rewritten, you can consider yourself now at a crossroads, able to decide which road to take. As you project forward to the future scene, then, practice taking the new road—visualize yourself being relaxed and confident in front of people, imagine yourself being able to be around flowers with your sinuses clear, imagine yourself eating only half the food on your plate and feeling quite satisfied, see yourself in a room full of people smoking with no desire to have a cigarette—and *really* experience this as you go through it.

You leave the relaxed state and come to full awakeness feeling comfortable and calm. You have a sense of having contacted some important material within yourself, and you have the feeling that there is a much better possibility for you to be the person that you really want to be in the future. The whole process has lasted about an hour.

I would at this point give you a cassette recording containing a relaxation procedure and suggestions for you to relive two or three similar memories and to rewrite them, followed by suggestions to project into the future and use image rehearsal of similar situations. My suggestion would be that you work with this tape two or three times a day, rewriting all the memories of this form that you can find—even ones we didn't get to during the session. You then develop creative, new solutions for these and practice handling more and more difficult situations in the future, always self-determining your behavior and your response. This allows your mind to build new expectations and adjusts and expands your self-image, clearing your mind of old patterns, increasing your creativity, and changing maladaptive responses. Practicing brings new confidence and courage in changing old ways.

The exploration you have just experienced is a very intense and vivid experience. In many ways, it is similar to going to a good play. Once you have entered the theatre or begun your exploration, all the usual daily problems, thoughts, distractions, and feelings are left outside; you focus on the stage, the players, and the scene at hand. You become very involved in each scene. In the case of the exploration, you are especially involved, because you are one of the main characters. All the time, you remain absorbed in the drama. You could become aware that you are in the theatre watching a play (or in the state of relaxation watching a memory), but you don't think about it—you become completely involved in the emotional quality and content of the action. When it is over, you do not forget;

you can recall everything that has happened. These memories remain available to you as you go about your daily activities.

Understanding on a deep level

After the exploration, you will have a series of memories involving emotions and bodily sensations. Their character and relationship to each other will allow you to understand how your maladaptive symptoms were created. How does it help to understand? The easiest way to demonstrate this is to use an example from advertising. The effects of advertising and its appeal to our subliminal nature disappear with insight and understanding. All you need to prove to yourself that a particular brand of shampoo is terrible is your own experience of using it. Once you have used it and found that you don't like it, all the advertising in the world meant to convince you that it's the "best" won't have any effect on you. You won't have to wonder whether or not you should use it; you know!

A story well known to students of behavioristic psychology demonstrates this point. A class of students decided to play a joke on their psychology professor. While he was lecturing, he had a habit of walking from one end of the classroom to the other. When he was in the left corner, the students smiled at him and were especially attentive. When he was in the right corner, they were noisy and fidgety. Before long, he had been positively conditioned to spend most of his lecture time in the left corner of the room. When the class told him what they had been doing, his behavior stopped. No amount of smiling would cause him to walk to the left side of the room. The insight and understanding of the situation allowed him to self-determine his behavior.

This story also demonstrates that even when we are teachers of the principles of conditioning we can still be programmed by the environment. Many of our maladaptive patterns are produced in a similar manner, and through awareness and understanding we can change. When you review in an exploration some of the actual events that have created your maladaptive patterns, an understanding takes place on many levels. First there is an intellectual understanding. This provides conscious knowledge that the story revealed "makes logical sense." In addition, there is an experiential understanding that involves the nonconscious part of the mind and the body. You have already experienced a new way of reacting. And all this has happened in a deeply relaxed state in which there is direct contact with the autonomic nervous system and extreme susceptibility to positive suggestion! It is like giving yourself a super-strong, experiential, posthypnotic suggestion to become the person you want to be . . . in the unique language of your own nonconscious mind.

Your role in the exploration is most important. Any sights or realizations gained from the experience will come from *you*—suggestions from a therapist serve as guides to lead you through the exploration. It's as if your natural healing abilities have been locked away, and these suggestions will provide the key that makes them available to you.

Generalization

When the mind is faced with a threatening circumstance, it will tend to react with the usual "fight–flight" response. As we have observed, the nonconscious mind remembers the situation so that if it arises again we can react from experience.

Perhaps you have heard the story of Albert, the infant who during a long hospital stay was noticed to cry and become cranky whenever he heard surgical instruments being clanked together. Albert had a furry, stuffed toy that he enjoyed caressing. On several occasions while Albert was touching his toy, he heard the sound of the instruments. Soon Albert refused to play with the toy, and eventually he cried whenever it was given to him. Though he was too young to make conscious choices, his nonconscious associated the surgical instruments and fear with his fuzzy animal. Before long, fear began to spread to other fuzzy toys, and before long Albert could not even tolerate fuzzy blankets. The survival value of generalization becomes clear when we recall our cave man ancestors and how we evolved—"it's better to be safe than sorry."

Similar observations can be made in adults. Do you ever experience anxiety when the phone rings, especially if it's at an odd hour, because you've received bad news over the phone in the past? The fear of finding out bad news is generalized to the ringing of the phone, and you may react even before knowing what the message is about. You may even react to the ringing of a phone in someone else's house. The man who is in a boating accident may generalize his discomfort to include all water—he refuses to sit by a swimming pool, take an ocean cruise, or walk along the beach.

The mind takes in stimuli through all the senses. If you're in a threatening situation, the mind will record sounds, smells, visual details of the surroundings, body position, feelings, and so on. In the future, if a similar threatening sound is heard, for instance, the body will react as if *all* the other cues were present. Imagine yourself in a mountain thunderstorm. It is hailing, lightning is flashing all around, and a tree is suddenly split by a bolt of lightning directly in front of you. You feel all the responses in your body that function to heighten your awareness so you can function effectively and get to safety. Years later, you again find yourself in a thunderstorm. It is simply a summer shower, but the first flash of lightning brings all the memories of the storm long ago. The mind tends to generalize the fear of certain objects or events to other *similar* objects or events in order to protect the organism from danger. Recall that Albert generalized his fear of his fuzzy toy to all fuzzy objects.

Imagine the dog who has a habit of digging bulbs out of gardens in the neighborhood. Yelling at him never does any good. One of the neighbors, Fred, decides to solve the problem. He decides to turn the hose on the dog, which sends him scampering off. The next day he's back in the garden, and Fred begins to pick up the hose. Before he can turn it on, the dog is gone. Several days later, the dog is in the yard again; but as Fred walks out the front door to chase him away, he runs off. A week later he is still digging up gardens at other houses in the neighborhood, but he doesn't go near Fred's property. The dog has generalized the fear of the hose, the sight of Fred, Fred's voice, and the scent of the whole yard; and so he stays completely away. If he is a very sensitive dog, he might begin to avoid all human contact.

This mechanism is a natural one that protects us from danger. It also points out a difficulty in tracing the roots of a physical symptom. It becomes very difficult to pinpoint the actual stimulus that caused the symptom to occur. Eventually, many different stimuli or perceptions can cause the same symptom or reaction. Similarly, one stimulus may trigger several reactions. After years of generalizing, it is almost impossible for the *conscious* mind to select specific causes, but the nonconscious mind *knows*; for *it is the nonconscious mind that makes the connections and creates the responses*. Our job then is to bring the knowledge of the nonconscious to consciousness so the patterns can be changed.

EDGAR

Edgar is a concert violinist who came in to explore a fear of being on stage. He had tried to use image visualization in the past to picture himself on stage without fear and had only limited success. He still experienced a stubborn knot of discomfort in his stomach that he couldn't seem to get rid of.

After relaxing through the use of selective awareness, he relived slowly and in detail several of the times in which he felt the fear. Through relaxation, his awareness was heightened, and Edgar discovered quite to his surprise that the stimulus responsible was *not playing* the violin in front of the audience; the fear actually coincided with the act of walking out in front of the audience carrying the violin. By reliving several memories in which he had felt this fear, Edgar realized that the fear began exactly at the moment he stepped from behind the curtain and out in front of the audience.

After recalling several more memories, I suggested that Edgar go back to the first time he experienced the fear. The sensitizing event occurred several years before his first concert when he was a young boy on his way to violin practice. He was surrounded by a group of older boys in the neighborhood who maliciously began to make fun of him for carrying a violin. He was told that if they ever saw him walking this way again, they would beat him up. He began to take back streets so he wouldn't be seen with his violin.

The act of *being seen with his violin* was the stimulus for fear in front of audiences.

Though he might have been able to recall some or all of these memories consciously, he had never connected them in this manner. In a state of deep relaxation, his mind brought out the specific details of a sensitizing event, which gave him new insight to his problem. Now he could consciously begin to adjust his self-image to deal specifically with walking out on stage with his violin and feeling comfortable and unafraid, since now he knew why his mind had begun the pattern; he had been threatened once for being seen with his violin, and his mind remembered it in order to warn him in similar situations in the future. After a few weeks of image rehearsal, entering the relaxed state, and visualizing successful performances, he was calmly playing in front of large audiences and enjoying it.[1]

Excessive fear and phobias

The so-called phobic responses provide us with some of the clearest examples of how we can involuntarily use our imagination to create mental pictures and then respond emotionally to them. A "phobia" is an exaggerated, inexplicable, and illogical fear of a specific object or a

---

[1]See Appendix. The cassette tape, "Changing Your Behavior Patterns—Writing Your Own Script," provides a way for an individual to begin to change his/her response patterns.

specific class of objects. Intense fear of an object or situation can be maladaptive and can create a state of imbalance. The most obvious characteristic of phobias is that they are extremely vivid. The image becomes so strongly imbedded in the mind that it is very difficult to change it by rational reasoning.

LYDIA

Lydia is a twenty-five-year-old woman who came in to explore her intense fear of water. Her husband and children were good swimmers, and they had just contracted to have a swimming pool built in their back yard. In the past, Lydia had dealt with her fear simply by avoiding water; but now she felt rather silly, since she couldn't even wade in the water up to her knees. Lydia "knew" why she was afraid of water—when she was very young she was told that it was possible to drown "in a teaspoon of water." When she was a small child, her mind responded to these words absolutely literally. Even though Lydia "knows" consciously why she has her irrational fear, her self-image is that water is dangerous to her and that she might drown if she goes near it. Lydia explained that she had tried to overcome her fear, but when she approached water she became so afraid that she would run away so she wouldn't become hysterical. She knows the fear is maladaptive, but she "can't help it."

Lydia decided to learn some methods of relaxation. She imagined herself going near the pool and walking down the steps into shallow water. The state of deep relaxation allowed her to imagine this without the overwhelming fear that she felt consciously when she went near the water. She imagined herself walking out into the water where she met her husband, who would teach her how to swim. She then imagined that all of this would take place that same afternoon when she was home.

Lydia finished the session and went home, only to call later
in the evening to report, "It happened just as I imagined it
would." She had used deep relaxation to change her self-
image from a woman "terrified of water" to a "swimmer
who is comfortable in the water." Her new self-image was
adaptive, and she no longer was threatened by the fear and
anxiety that created a state of imbalance in her life. After
several seeks she confidently reported a complete and
permanent "cure."

Let's look at an example where the *cause* of the fear is not
obvious.

SALLY

Sally is a homemaker who lives in San Francisco. She had a
tremendous fear of bridges, which posed quite a problem
for her when it came to traveling to the communities surrounding the city of San Francisco. Her fear of bridges
began to affect her life when she refused to attend social
events with her husband in the Bay Area when it required
crossing a bridge.

Sally came in for an exploration and discovered that her
fear of bridges was merely a symptom of a deeper fear—
fear of her mother's criticism of her and fear of failure.
Every time she visited her mother, Sally felt defeated,
ridiculed, and very much a failure. Her mother disap-
proved of her marriage, her lifestyle, and of the way she
was raising her children. In order to reach her mother's
house, Sally had to cross the Golden Gate Bridge! She always felt tense and anxious crossing the bridge, anticipat-
ing the interaction with her mother; yet she felt obligated
to visit her and put up with the unpleasantness. Her nonconscious mind began to react to the tension in her body as
she crossed the bridge. Before long she could not bring

herself to drive across it or even to be driven across it—her fear gave her a reason not to visit her mother! Soon the process of generalization resulted in an irrational fear response to all bridges.

Through an exploration, Sally realized that her fear of bridges was maladaptive. She also understood the roots of the problem. She began to change the image she had of herself as a failure, and soon she was not only crossing bridges but was able to be more realistic about her mother's criticism and not take it so seriously.

As we move to symptoms and problems that are expressed primarily through physical rather than emotional channels, it becomes even more fascinating for us to see how our minds and bodies respond to fears or situations. We'll see how explorations can elucidate the causes of physical symptoms that on the surface seem unrelated to emotions.

11
Old symptoms and new cures

The one-eyed doe

A doe who had had the misfortune to lose the sight of one of her eyes, and so could not see anyone approaching on that side, made it her practice to graze on a high cliff near the sea. Thus she kept her good eye toward the land on the lookout for hunters, while her blind side was toward the sea whence she feared no danger.

But one day some sailors were rowing past in a boat. Catching sight of the doe as she was grazing peacefully along the edge of the cliff, one of the sailors drew his bow and shot her. With her last gasp the dying doe said: "Alas, ill-fated creature that I am! I was safe on the land side, whence I looked for danger, but my enemy came from the sea, to which I looked for protection."

APPLICATION: Trouble comes from the direction we least expect it.

141

The common cold

Physicians ordinarily treat colds with nasal decongestants, antihistamines, throat lozenges, cough syrups, vitamin supplements, and the like; a large variety of "home remedies" are also common. But the common cold is viral and therefore unresponsive to antibiotics—it must run its course while we "grin and bear it."

If we look more closely at the common cold, we find that some people seem to "catch" colds often, whereas others rarely or never are bothered with them. Every day doctors see patients with infections ranging from the sniffles, sore throats, and coughs to full-blown cases of pneumonia. In almost every case, the patient believes that he or she has "caught" the cold from someone else. One of the major modes of spreading infection is through coughing and sneezing; the germs are transmitted through the air and inhaled by others. It should follow, then, that doctors get colds much more frequently than others who are not exposed to germs all the time. Such is not the case. This leads us to consider that the susceptibility of the patient is often a more significant factor in the development of the cold than the infectiousness of the viral or bacterial organism itself. This susceptibility is often the result of an imbalance in the body that has been produced by a change in emotional or physical conditions. IMBALANCE LEADS TO INCREASED SUSCEPTIBILITY TO DISEASE!

With every breath, we take in air laden with bacteria and viruses of many types. One of the main functions of the cells of the throat is to moisten and clean the air to prevent infection. Generally these defense mechanisms are quite effective, but occasionally they break down. To assume that the presence of microorganisms is the whole cause for the breakdown of these defense mechanisms is incorrect. Some people carry bacteria and viruses for months with no signs of an infection whatsoever. Here again we see that each of us has a unique way of responding to infectious agents in the environment, depending on our own specific conditions.

SAM

Sam came in complaining of a sore throat, a high temperature, and swollen lymph nodes in his neck. Streptococcal bacteria were found in his throat during the examination, and his pharynx was red and inflamed. Sam's defense mechanisms had broken down. We discussed some of the events of Sam's life during the past few days that might have caused his increased susceptibility to germs.

Sam thought back a few days before the sore throat developed and remembered an incident that still bothered him—he had lost a brief case full of some important papers that belonged to the insurance company where he worked. This was not Sam's first mistake; he had been warned before about his unreliability. Sam decided that telling the truth was too much of a risk, so he told his boss that he had left the brief case on the desk of one of his coworkers and didn't know what happened to them after that. The office was searched, but no papers were found. Sam's coworkers were frustrated and perplexed, but the blame could not be placed on Sam. Sam could *not*, however, escape from the tension and anxiety he felt as he told people that he didn't know where the papers were.

The inconsistency in Sam's story created an imbalance in his body. His emotional anxiety became maladaptive, and for the next few days he felt unhappy and uncomfortable. Though he may not have been aware of it, there was a good deal of tension around the area of his vocal cords and throat. The streptococci, which may have been in Sam's throat for a long time, now began to grow in this area that was more susceptible due to tension. With the imbalance that Sam had created in his body, his throat was a perfect target for a physical symptom. Once the germs had multiplied, other complications such as pain in the joints and fever were likely to occur. Now Sam needed medication to help his natural defense system restore balance. If the pattern of protecting himself by lying in this way should become habitual, Sam might end up with repeated, chronic sore throats and colds.

Sam's case is one example of how physical tension and emotional anxiety can upset the balance and produce organic disease. Somehow changes in the mind are ultimately translated into cellular and molecular change. Some people will develop a cold or sore throat several days before a speaking engagement. Others often develop a cold or other physical problem just before a vacation that has been planned for months. So anxious are these people that the vacation be "perfect" they often can't even enjoy it. Can you think of any similar examples in your life?

Of course, every bacterial infection is not necessarily the result of this process of lowered resistance. Some germs may even be strong enough to overcome the defense mechanisms of even the well-balanced system— measles, plague, and smallpox, for example. Differences in genetic characteristics, nutritional state, and general physical condition also help determine susceptibility.

Next time you find yourself with a cold or a respiratory infection, consider the events just prior to the development of your symptoms—specific tensions at work, school, with your family; decisions that were uncomfortable to make, arguments with friends, and so on. Most people discover that they can clearly point to events that may have precipitated their symptoms. This added understanding, along with the appropriate medication, seems to alleviate the symptoms more quickly. We can refer to our discussion of the self-image to explain this. Once you have *accepted* the behavior that may have made you tense and anxious and can form a realistic means of dealing with it, you no longer have to carry the tension around with you to other areas of your life where it may be maladaptive. And without tension and anxiety, the healing processes are accelerated, and balance is restored more quickly.

HARRY

Harry is an attorney. Several times a year he found himself with a cold or the flu, accompanied by muscle pains, backaches, tiredness, and fever. When the symptoms occurred, Harry was forced to take a week off to stay in bed. Lately, he'd been feeling more and more upset with these episodes of the flu—he'd been losing money, was tired of staying home in bed, and was using up his vacation time with sick leave. Harry came to see me for help with this problem, and I suggested we try an exploration to find the source of his recurring symptoms. After he was deeply relaxed, I suggested he go back to the day before his body first began to experience the imbalance that led to his most recent illness.

. . . Harry drifted back a few days before to a day when he was at work with a long schedule ahead. It was a beautiful day outside, and he was wishing he didn't have to work so hard; he felt uncomfortable and restless. . . . The next morning he woke up with the flu.

Harry recalled a series of memories during the past years where he'd been in similar situations—working hard and having no time off. He then recalled the sensitizing event.

. . . Harry was a young boy in the fifth grade. On the next day at school he had an important spelling test. He wanted to do well, and his parents expected him to get an "A." He felt anxious and unhappy; he hadn't studied and wished he weren't under so much pressure. The next morning, Harry's mother came in to wake him for school and discovered that he had the measles. Harry greeted the news with relief! He was happy to stay home sick and avoid failing the spelling exam. . . .

Harry had begun a pattern of getting sick in the midst of pressure and uncomfortable situations when he felt trapped by his responsibilities. His nonconscious mind, when it felt too much pressure, simply allowed his resistance to drop to the point where one of the viruses in the environment could invade his body and provide an escape from tension.

Following the exploration, Harry could see his problem clearly. He realized that he had always had an image of himself always working, always obligated, always under pressure, and always tired. Taking time off would be admitting failure—that he had let himself down. Harry realized that this aspect of his self-image was maladaptive.

He began to plan occasional three-day weekends and short trips. In the months that followed he had no further episodes of colds and flu. Harry also noticed a change in the quality of his life. He no longer dreaded an exhausting schedule. Once he'd learned how to restore his balance when he was fatigued and overworked, he no longer had to feel tense and anxious about a busy schedule.

Several years have passed, and Harry is hardly ever sick. The biggest problem now is that of his secretary. Harry sometimes gets the idea that he needs a rest and suddenly calls in and tells her to cancel all his appointments for two days!

Allergies

Allergies are widespread in our culture, and medical literature indicates that man has suffered from them for centuries. Traditional treatment for allergic reactions has been to remove the substance that seems to cause the trouble from the environment of the patient or to administer medication that prevents the body from responding to the substance.

There are probably millions of different, specific molecules that we may become allergic to. You may know someone who is allergic to cat fur but not dog fur; walnuts but not peanuts, roses but not daffodils. Allergies are most often determined by skin testing. Skin testing is performed by injecting small amounts of various proteins under the skin. Those injection sites that show redness, swelling, and itching indicate the protein to which the person has become allergic. The swelling and redness are produced primarily through the action of histamine—a chemical released from certain body cells when an allergic reaction is taking place in that area. Antihistamines are often prescribed to diminish the symptoms of allergies. Why does the body choose only a certain set of molecules to react against and ignore others? And why is it that humans have so many more problems with allergies than other animals?

Human beings are perhaps the only animals who will stay around in an unpleasant situation—one of the effects

of socialization. At work, in school, on the freeway, or in
the midst of an argument we stand still and accumulate
levels of tension that would send any other self-respecting
animal fleeing for safety. We have many ways of justifying
our behavior—social manners, pride, pressure from
others, fear of punishment, and so on. The decision to
remain in a situation of fear and high tension is a conscious
one; we believe that we understand what we are doing.
The nonconscious mind, however, still functions as if our
survival is threatened ("fight or flight") and looks to find
an explanation for the fear and anxiety we are feeling.
The nonconscious mind reasons that the tension couldn't
be the result of the *external* situation, or else we would be
running away; the physiological signs that would dictate
"fight–flight" behavior are present, yet nothing is happening. When we do nothing to alleviate the tension (like fight
or flight, the natural animal reaction), the mind reasons
that it must be under attack by something else— something *internal*.

　　The body's way of responding to internal attacks by
foreign molecules is to form antibodies against them.
When the foreign molecules are those of either a virus or
bacteria, the antibodies serve to inactivate them and also
act as a "tag" that attracts white blood cells. The white
blood cells can then gobble up the particles and carry them
away. In the case of allergies, however, the foreign
molecules are actually *not* a threat to the body, and nature
has not provided a mechanism for completely inactivating
them.

　　In a situation of stress from which we do not flee, it
may be that by coincidence a certain foreign protein is
present in the body. The nonconscious mind may decide

that this protein is dangerous and try to get rid of it in the usual manner. The body can only form "incomplete" antibodies (haptens) for these proteins; i.e., the antibody only partially combines with the foreign substance, and the resulting molecule is an irritant that causes histamine to be released, which in turn produces the allergic symptoms.

Imagine the child who is being scolded. He may be extremely frightened but doesn't leave or fight back, because that would result in more unpleasant consequences. The nonconscious responds to the fear as though it were an actual threat to survival. It reasons that since the child is not running away, the tension must be from inside the body and it begins to search for the source of the threat; the nonconscious mind may discover some walnut molecues on the lining of the oral cavity and tongue and decide that they are the cause of the tension. His body attempts to attack these proteins. The incomplete antibodies result in an inflammatory reaction in the body, characterized by the tissues becoming hot and swollen. His tongue and mouth get red, and they begin to hurt. An allergic response is started. In a few weeks if the child should eat walnuts, he may react as before, even if there is no emotional stress. His mind "remembers" the amount of tension and the fear, and his allergic reaction is activated (the anamnestic response). His mouth and tongue are the target organs. In a like manner, when he gets upset in an emotional situation, his allergic symptoms may flare up!

The usual treatments for allergies are prescriptions for antihistamines to decrease the swelling of the mucous membranes or hydrocortisone, which prevents the body from reacting to the foreign substance. Both of these treatments are symptomatic, and the allergy remains. Ex-

ploration, desensitization, and positive imagery can often
be used effectively to find the emotional source of an allergy and eliminate it permanently.

Bob

Bob had suffered from hay fever for many years, and it
had become so severe that he was unable to drive past a
field of hay without uncomfortable symptoms—nasal con-
gestion, itching eyes, and tears. In an exploration, Bob recalled memories that led to his allergic symptoms. In each
memory he was passing a field of hay. Bob then recalled
the sensitizing event—the first time in his life that the allergic reaction had taken place:

... Bob was three years old. His father asked him if he
would like to visit his grandfather in the country. He recalled sitting next to his father in the car and riding past
fields and farmhouses. He remembered bales of hay piled
up in the yard of his grandfather's house and a red tractor.
Standing next to the tractor was a man in grey overalls
wearing a huge, cylindrical, metal mask; his face was covered with a glass plate. In his hand was a long wire attached
to a machine that was making a tremendous amount of
noise. At the end of the wire was a blinding bright light.
Bob recalled the fear he felt as he cried and hid from the
"monster" on the floor of the car. All his relatives were
laughing at him, and he felt ashamed. His father pulled
him from the car to bring him closer to the tractor, urging
him to be a man and stop crying. He was terrified. . . . At
that point in the exploration, Bob was crying and began to
experience the symptoms of his allergy.

Many people who are exploring patterns involving physical
symptoms experience the onset of the symptom during
certain memories (abreaction).

After he had once again become completely relaxed, Bob could understand that what he had seen as a child was a welder working on the tractor. Until the exploration, he had absolutely no memory of the incident. Now he could see how his body had misunderstood the tension and fear and chosen the hay as the source. The hay proteins had been on his mucous membranes when his nonconscious mind looked around for the source of the threat. Bob had built two maladaptive aspects into his self-image: Hay was dangerous and threatening, and people laughed at him when he was afraid. Once he understood how this happened and saw that it was not adaptive, he could build a more realistic image of himself. And his hay fever disappeared!

Many people have solved their allergy problems through such processes as the exploration. In each case, a situation(s) of high emotional tension was associated with the contact of a specific part of the body to a foreign substance. Of course, not everyone with a high degree of tension in a hay field will develop an allergy. Whether or not this occurs depends on the unique responses, genetic tendencies, and physiological makeup of each one of us.

The endocrine system

Diseases associated with the endocrine system range from diabetes to an overactive thyroid to irregular menstrual periods to "hypoglycemia." The system consists of many glands that empty their chemical products (hormones) directly into the blood stream. Endocrine glands include the thyroid gland, the parathyroids, the pineal gland, the pituitary gland, the sexual glands, the pancreas, and the adrenal glands. The endocrine glands govern nearly every aspect of body functioning, including metabolism, sugar usage, levels of muscular tension, sexual functioning, and moods; and they are important in maintaining proper homeostatic balance. The endocrine organs are like massively developed nerve endings that produce hormones which cause changes in the body in much the same way as all other nerves do. These hormones circulate through the blood stream and are the means by which the body makes gross adjustments to the environment. The ouput of the adrenals, for instance, is necessary at times of stress ("fight–flight" response). The release of adrenalin and the resulting rapid breathing and pounding heart that you feel in a situation of anxiety and fear is an endocrine function.

The endocrine system is closely associated with the nervous system and like the nervous system responds to the influences of emotions. We may secrete too much or too little hormone, thus creating an imbalance in the body. This imbalance may be caused by factors in the environment, the self-image, or emotional responses. People have reported improvements in glandular functioning after using relaxation processes to adjust the self-image through the imagination.

The interruption of the normal patterns of an endocrine gland can become the roots of a future dysfunction.

BETTY

Betty came in to explore why she wasn't losing weight after weeks of strict dieting. She also complained of feeling tired and sluggish most of the time.

When Betty was a young child her parents became angry with her whenever she played noisily. Her mother would come in and put her to bed whenever she became active. As this became a repeated pattern, Betty began associating active play and self expression with a high degree of tension—tension created when her parents would scold her for being too noisy.

The thyroid gland controls the overall body activity, and after several years of this repeated pattern, Betty became "less active" in response to the way she was treated. She had built a self-image that it was *wrong* to be active, and she was always afraid of being punished. One way the body generally carries out the command to become less active is to decrease the output of the thyroid hormone. By the time Betty was in high school she was sluggish and overweight and had a hypothyroid condition.

After an exploration Betty realized how her mind had distorted the incidents in her childhood. Until this time she had been on diet after diet, only to feel frustrated and discouraged when she was unsuccessful. As she began to readjust her self-image to be more adaptive Betty began to lose weight gradually and steadily. Her discouragement over feeling tired also disappeared as she realized that she would no longer be punished for being active and energetic, and she no longer had to carry the tension associated with that fear. She also experienced a diminished need for thyroid hormone pills.

Imagine the common situation of parents who punish their children for exploring or even asking about their sexual organs or their functions. This brings about the association of tension, fear, and anxiety with the sexual glands and the sex organs. It's easy to see how in later life many of us have difficulties in our marriage and sexual relationships: pain during intercourse, nonresponsiveness, guilt or fear about sexual feelings, troublesome periods, inability to express love, so-called impotence, problems with childbirth, and so on. Breast development is also dependent upon the normal functioning of the sexual glands. Delayed breast development can occur as a function of the association of the breasts or sexual organs with fear and anxiety.

A common example of the close and often dramatic connection between moods and feelings and the functioning of the endocrine system is the young woman who misses her menstrual period by one, two, or three weeks. Finally she has a pregnancy test performed, and upon finding she is not pregnant she begins her period that very day. The tension has been relieved, the fear of being pregnant is gone, and the glands function normally again! Similarly, the woman who has tried for years to become pregnant finally adopts a child—then becomes pregnant the next month because she is no longer tense and trying.

Skin problems

The skin is the largest single organ in the body. It goes through a wide range of reactions due to emotional changes, including the release of perspiration, blushing, common rashes, hives, blisters, itching, redness, soreness, and breakdown of tissue.

Often there is no offending bacterium or virus in skin problems. They often seem to appear from "unknown" causes. In many people with skin problems, I have found the explorations seem to indicate that the body is attacking

its own tissue overresponding to a minor irritation or causing irritation to itself in some way.

One of the most common treatments for skin problems is cortisone: cream, tablets, or injections. Cortisone is
a chemical produced by the endocrine system that partially
paralyzes the body's ability to respond to irritants and
foreign invaders. Thus there are dangers in giving a patient larger amounts than the body is producing. They
must be carefully checked for tuberculosis, for example,
before the drug is administered; once cortisone is given
dormant organisms seem to gain new life and penetrate
the body's defenses. If we hypothesize that a skin condition
is in some way a self-attack, we can imagine how cortisone
provides relief by blocking the body's ability to train its
defensive forces on itself!

A large number of skin problems seem to appear on
the face. Many people with facial blemishes are highly
self-conscious and easily embarrassed by anything that is
not "just so" on their bodies. It seems unfortunate indeed
that these people have an unsightly condition on the one
part of their body that everyone can see—the one part they
cannot hide in social situations. As we have observed with
other physical symptoms, perhaps more than "bad luck" is
involved.

MARJORIE

Marjorie came in requesting cortisone for an unsightly skin
condition of her face. She had been suffering from this
problem on and off for several years. She was deeply embarrassed and unhappy with her blemishes.

As a child, Marjorie was taught to be very conscious of her

appearance. Weeks before her first high school dance, she began to fear that something would go wrong. One day while looking in the mirror, she noticed a small, red mark on her face. She reacted with tears, anger, discouragement, and fear that she would not be able to go to the dance. Over the next couple of weeks her rash got worse, and her worst expectation came true. She felt miserable about having to stay home from this important event.

In the years that followed, whenever Marjorie was especially anxious or nervous about an interview, a meeting, or a party, the rash would reappear. Her self-consciousness began to get worse and worse.

After an exploration, Marjorie began to see how she had built feelings of inadequacy and embarrassment into her self-image. She realized that her physical symptoms were a way to escape. She used the rash to stay home from any event where she might feel anxious and uncomfortable. She began to clearly see that the circumstances in her life that made her unhappy were a reflection of the image she had of herself ("you are what you think you are").

Marjorie learned that her anxiety over her skin problem and her self-consciousness was maladaptive. She began to practice relaxation processes each day and started imagining herself in situations where she was at ease with people; she began to smile at her face in the mirror, relieving the emotional tension and accepting the rash in a relaxed manner. As her self-image adjusted itself to a more adaptive balance, the rash began to disappear.

Vision—the eyes have it, too

Like most people, I had always assumed that nearsightedness and farsightedness were basically inherited or structural problems that were permanent in an individual's life. I was accustomed to the standard treatment—a prescription of lenses to bring the rays of light to focus at the right point on the retina. This belief changed dramatically for me in one single week.

It was in my early days of practicing hypnosis, and I was fascinated by the effects that suggestion could have on normally nonconscious processes. One day I was exploring the possibilities of hypnosis with a subject, teaching him how to cause the size of his pupils to change merely through suggestion. He then asked me whether or not it was possible to affect his visual acuity. As his vision was 20/100 in one eye, I naturally assumed that he wanted to correct his vision. He quickly informed me, however, that he was interested in seeing whether or not it was possible, through suggestion, to temporarily change his vision so that it would be 20/400 in this eye. I thought it was a strange request, but I agreed to do so and placed him in front of an eye chart. By moving him from twenty feet, to fifteen feet, and then to ten feet while giving him suggestions that he would be able to see only the appropriate line on the eye chart in focus, he soon seemed to learn this feat. Following the experiment, he was able to return his vision in this eye to 20/100; he did so and left.

I didn't see him for another three weeks, at which time he stopped by my office, smiling and waving a piece of paper in his hand. "Thanks, Doc! Now I don't have to go to Vietnam!" I questioned him further about this; and he told me that with his vision 20/100 in that eye, he was still eligible for the draft, which was then in force due to the unpopular conflict in Vietnam. As he was strongly opposed to being in the Army at this time, he had made me his unwitting accomplice and avoided being drafted by giving himself the suggestion to change his vision for the worst while at his draft physical.

He described to me how he had been sent to an ophthalmologist, who dilated his pupils and put various lenses in front of his eyes. Even under this careful testing, the lens of his eye still behaved as though he were much more nearsighted than was actually the case. He was rejected; and as he left the induction center, he happily reversed his suggestion, his eyesight went back to what it had always been, and he was able to drive home. As I watched him climb into his homemade camper and leave for an extended camping trip in the desert, I realized that I had just learned another lesson about the remarkably intimate contact between the human mind and body.

Some visual disorders may be linked to highly emotional sensitizing events. Many people who wear glasses may be aware of fluctuations in their visual acuity in different emotional situations. These people who are aware of their vision changing occasionally in relation to their moods probably stand the best chance of improving it through relaxation and imagery.

Let's look at the case of Tommy, a two-year-old boy who is taken to the zoo by his parents for an afternoon visit. It's a warm, sunny day, and Tommy falls asleep against his mother's shoulder while they are passing the lion's cage. The lion, playing in the cage with his mates, soon lets out a deafening roar. Tommy is startled, and when his eyes open he sees the lion's gaping jaws and is terrified. As he turns his head and sees his mother, the level of tension begins to decrease, and he feels safe. Once he feels safe, he cautiously begins to peek over his mother's shoulder to look again at the frightening animal and then quickly focuses on his mother for reassurance. Each time his eyes are focused on the lion, he feels tension; when he quickly changes his focus to look at his mother, he feels a release of tension; i.e., he feels tension when gazing at an object in the distance and relaxation when he focuses on something close to him. As Tommy grows older, he experiences similar events, and he notices that when he is very frightened or angry, his vision seems to blur. His mother takes him to an ophthalmologist. Tommy finds out that he is nearsighted (unable to see distant objects clearly), and corrective lenses are prescribed.

Children often begin to need glasses during the years of puberty, when stress, social pressure, and challenge outside the home are heightened. Tension and fear may cause the classroom blackboard to "slip into blurriness." Certainly this is not the case with all visual problems or even with most of them. It has been found, however, that many people when in a state of deep relaxation can see perfectly well without their glasses or find that vision is considerably improved. As in Tommy's case, a person with visual defects may find the sensitizing events or series of sensitizing events that caused them to create an image of "being afraid to see clearly." By readjusting the self-image, these people have been able to watch their vision gradually and steadily improve until some have been able to throw their glasses away!

Dr. William Bates has devoted his career to similar concepts. In his book, *Better Eyesight Without Glasses* (Holt, Rinehart and Winston, New York, 1943), he discusses methods of eye exercise and mental relaxation that he has developed that have resulted in amazing cures. Bates believes that changes in the eye that produce nearsightedness and farsightedness are not necessarily permanent. His work indicates that relaxing and rebalancing the eye muscles can lead to improvement in vision. The Bates method has many principles that are similar to the ones we've been discussing.

Surgery

In medicine, there is a condition known as the "gridiron" abdomen syndrome. This syndrome refers to the presence of certain multiple abdominal operations (exploratory surgery, removal of gall bladder, appendix, ulcers, and so on). The term "gridiron" describes the surgical scars that crisscross each other. For many persons having this syndrome, daily tension and anxieties are expressed through pathological changes in the abdominal organs; and imbalances are created. The imbalances often disrupt muscles and glands and cause circulatory and digestive problems. The "gridiron" syndrome represents an extreme case, but it illustrates how maladaptive tensions can lead to surgery. In many cases, it may be possible to control problems that would usually lead to surgery with relaxation rather than with the traditional painful, expensive, and time-consuming surgical procedures and lengthy recovery periods.

JOAN

Joan had had surgery several times in the last twenty years. She came in with a feeling of desperation, as she was again faced with the prospect of hospitalization—her physician had suggested exploratory surgery for an intractable pain in the abdomen. She was also having some problems in her marriage. In an exploration, she worked her way back to an early sensitizing event:

. . . Joan was six years old and in the first grade. On the way home from school one day, she stopped to pick some green apples from a neighbor's tree, which she then ate. By the time she got home, Joan had quite a stomach-ache. When she ran into her parents' room, she surprised them in the midst of an argument. They were embarrassed and angrily told her that she deserved to have the stomach-ache—that it would teach her not to pick fruit and eat it without first checking to see if it was safe. Joan felt lonely, rejected, and hurt. As she went to her room to lie on her bed, she still felt the severe pain in her stomach.

Here we see a situation where high emotional tension is associated with physical tension in the abdominal organs. This was the beginning of a pattern in Joan's life. As she grew older she had occasional stomach-aches as all children do, but she tended to always feel anxious and afraid during these times. This anxiety further increased the spasm and delayed healing, and her stomach-aches became more and more serious. She also began to notice that feelings of rejection, loneliness, or guilt would cause her stomach to "knot up." When she argued with people, she would feel a similar sensation in her stomach. Sometimes she even had the eerie feeling that she "deserved this pain."

In later years, Joan underwent an appendectomy, a hysterectomy, and surgery for an ulcer. In each case, similar feelings of rejection, loneliness, and anxiety occurred in a relationship with someone she loved in the weeks immediately prior to the surgery.

Joan felt that she could not bear to have another operation—the stress and strain of surgery and hospitalization were becoming too painful. She started working on relaxing the muscles in her abdomen. She realized that she felt the worst pains when she was afraid that her husband would leave her. Looking back through the memories that came up for her in the exploration, she realized how she had always associated rejection with pain in her stomach; she began to see how this was maladaptive.

Each day Joan practiced relaxation, using imagery to picture her internal organs relaxing. She then replayed those disappointing periods in her life, this time rewriting her script, imagining that she was going through them with a relaxed body. Daily she experienced a decrease in the anxiety and tension and the pain in her abdomen. It gradually began to fade away as the deeper levels of her mind realized how the pattern had been created and that it was maladaptive. Before long she felt much stronger physically and no longer had to face the possibility of surgery—her abdominal pain had disappeared! Theses new changes in her life gave her courage to face the problems with her husband.

Again I want to make it clear that not all surgical problems can be solved outside the operating room. Certainly the patient with a ruptured appendix needs immediate surgery. So, also, may the patient in severe pain need hospitalization and exploratory surgery. We can now, however, take preventive measures with potential surgical problems, so that the physical imbalance underlying the symptoms can be eliminated before surgery becomes the only recourse.

Even in cases where surgery is necessary, relaxation processes allow the person to handle the experience with more ease and with less pain and anxiety during recovery. With relaxation processes, you can create the environment in which your healing abilities can function maximally. Surgeons have found complications such as pain and infection much less common when patients have been taught these processes beforehand.

MARTHA

Martha was facing an operation for cataracts. This surgery for her, however, was especially dangerous. She had a lung problem and was unable to undergo general anesthesia; deep levels of anesthesia made it dangerously difficult for her to breath. Under lighter levels of anesthesia, Martha had a problem with coughing, making the delicate procedures for eye surgery impossible. She came in to explore another way to have the surgery performed.

Martha first learned the processes of deep relaxation. While she was relaxed, she began to practice focusing on her breathing to keep it constant, rhythmic, and steady. She went through an "imaginary" surgery where she was told every step that would happen. During this procedure she was deeply relaxed and continued to be aware of her breathing. She realized that her coughing problem represented the fear she experienced facing surgery. As she gained confidence about the procedure, she was able to inhibit the cough through relaxation and autosuggestion. On the day of the surgery, she felt confident and relaxed; there was no coughing to interrupt the surgeon; her surgery was successful and her recovery period short!

A maladaptive aspect of the self-image can create serious postoperative problems and delay normal healing. Likewise, adjusting the self-image through the use of relaxation and imagination can create an environment where the problems can clear up.

TODD

Todd is a young man who was injured in the war. During a battle, he was hit in the leg, and a chunk of metal was embedded there. Todd's only thought was, "I'll never walk again"—no sports, no jogging on the beach, no dancing, and so forth. He had overwhelming feelings of fear, despair, and sadness as he thought of himself crippled and in a wheel chair for the rest of his life. He lost consciousness and awoke following surgery in a field hospital. His leg had been amputated just below the knee, and the doctors expected adequate function with a prosthesis (artificial leg). Unfortunately, this was not the case. Using a prosthesis caused Todd great pain, and the skin over the operated area kept breaking down. Soon he was confined to a wheel chair.

Todd was growing more depressed and becoming increasingly dependent on pain medication. He was referred to me by his surgeon, who felt a psychosomatic problem might be preventing the normal response in this healthy man. We decided to do an exploration to look for the roots of his problem. Many of his memories were filled with helpless, hopeless despair. The image Todd held of himself was that of a helpless cripple. He traced his memories back to the sensitizing event. This was an event in Todd's childhood when he witnessed a group of boys making fun of another child who was unable to walk as a result of polio. The sorrow and hopelessness he felt had caused him to begin to associate being crippled with intense fear and sadness. Later in life when he was faced with the prospect of being crippled, the feelings of hopelessness resurfaced.

By using his imagination to recreate his memories with a more adaptive attitude, Todd's self-image began to adjust itself. He no longer had to see himself as a helpless cripple. Within weeks he was off pain medication and was walking comfortably on his prosthesis.

Pregnancy and childbirth

Tension, anxiety, and pain are often significant causes of complications during pregnancy and childbirth. The common fears associated with doctors, hospitals, scalpels, the labor and delivery injections, intravenous fluids, and anesthesia are often present during childbirth. It is curious that our culture creates the same hospital-type environment for the natural process of childbirth as it does for serious pathologies and complicated surgery. In our culture, many women have been taught to "fear" childbirth. Excruciating pain is *not* an essential part of the process. In births utilizing hypnosis. Lamaze, and other similar relaxation techniques, many women report *no* pain.

Here we see the effect of the "self-image" many American women have. Women are constantly presented with photographs, stories, and newspaper items of deformed children, the dangers of contraceptives and fertility drugs, and of deaths due to pregnancy. Even the natural, uterine contractions that occur during birth are called labor "pains" in our culture. Women hear stories of the vaginal tissue tearing during childbirth, requiring painful surgery to repair. With all our modern skills in obstetrics, physicians have often failed to pass on to expectant mothers and fathers the information that the mother's own tension and fear can cause the pain and complications during childbirth. A woman who is frightened when the infant's head begins to emerge is much more likely to tear her vaginal tissue with a panic-stricken "push" rather than to allow the process to continue smoothly and slowly.

As we have observed, we can eliminate tension and fear that is maladaptive. Many women have learned to experience "natural childbirth." The techniques focus on eliminating fear and substituting positive expectations that allow both the mother and the father to have a joyful experience during childbirth. Methods of relaxation are taught, along with breathing exercises that encourage slow, smooth, constant breathing. Rapid, irregular breathing causes changes in the body that tend to increase muscular tension and anxiety.

By using relaxation and imagination, women can begin to realize that pregnancy and delivery are natural functions and that the muscular contractions of the uterus need be no more painful than the contractions of the biceps muscle or of any other muscle in the body. The use of these processes can also lead to the quick return of strength and normal functioning for the mother. The emotional state of the mother has profound implications for the health of the child; when the mother is relaxed and calm during delivery, the child is less likely to be in distress and have complications during the birth process. In the future, we may decide to stop using the word "labor" to describe contractions as we begin to realize that childbirth is *nonlabor*; it's a matter of allowing the process to occur naturally. Proper contractions occur as automatically and as naturally as the heartbeat.

There is now excellent evidence that we store our birth experience in our nonconscious minds. Some people have experienced lifelong feelings of rejection and loneliness dating back to being carried by a cold, unfriendly nurse shortly after birth. It makes more sense to allow the child to be with the parents as much as possible. It also makes sense to dim the lights in the delivery room, to ask attendants to be relaxed and pleasant, and to refrain from using such words as "pain," "hurt," "shot," and other expressions that imply discomfort and disability. The reason for dimming the lights stems from the results of many explorations that led back to the birth experience and the trauma of bright lights shining on masked faces.

GAIL

Gail is a young woman who feared pregnancy and delivery. She and her husband had decided that they wanted a child; and she came in to explore her fears, which she realized were maladaptive. In an exploration, Gail remembered being told stories of the terrible pain of childbirth when she was a child. She also recalled an intense fear of her sexual organs during her developmental years. While in a state of deep relaxation, Gail recalled her birth experience:

She recalled the feelings of pressure on her head and the sounds of her mother screaming as she was being pulled out the birth canal. She could even describe the surgical clamps on her head, the dazzling white lights, the clanking of surgical instruments and the feelings of panic and confusion. As the doctor held her, she felt wet and cold; and she recalled the words, "Oh, no, not another girl!"

After the exploration, Gail discussed her memories. She had always known that her mother had a great fear of pain; now she realized how deeply ingrained the experience had become in her own life. She also realized how her mother's disappointment at her birth came about. All of her aunts had given birth to girls, and her grandfather and father desperately wanted a boy. Gail had several more sessions where she relived these memories and allowed her self-image to adjust itself and diminish her fear of pregnancy. She practiced relaxation processes for several weeks and was happily looking forward to becoming pregnant. . . .

During the last month of her pregnancy, Gail was taught hypnoanesthesia. She practiced by imagining herself relaxed and comfortable during delivery, while the natural uterine contractions occurred. She went through delivery without difficulty. She was wide awake and smiling. She

167

had a minor tear in the vaginal tissue, which was sutured without anesthesia while she held the baby. After her own experience of birth, which she had become aware of during her exploration, she realized the importance of her baby's first few minutes. She experienced the joy of being relaxed and having her husband at her side and said to her child, "What a beautiful baby; you'll grow up strong, healthy, and happy!"

Stress diseases

High blood pressure, heart disease, arthritis, and tremors that often occur as we grow older are often called the diseases of aging or the *stress* diseases. We are generally not surprised to see these disorders develop as people grow to maturity. Very seldom is anything done to find the source of these problems. As in most other cases, treatment tends to be symptomatic. These diseases commonly get worse with time and often lead to premature death. We are now beginning to see that many of these problems can be prevented, ameliorated, or even cured with the processes we've been discussing. How different our culture would be if we could approach old age with the attitude that we can maintain good physical health and emotional balance!

The prevention of these diseases may be accomplished by beginning to eliminate emotional tensions *now*, before the development of serious physical symptoms becomes inevitable. Even if the symptoms have already occurred, you might be able to keep them from progressing any further or possibly eliminate them altogether.

JOHN

John, a man in his early fifties, has angina pectoris. Angina pectoris is a pain produced by lack of oxygen in the heart muscle and is usually caused by blockages in the coronary arteries. It is similar to the cramps in other musles that result from stress on the muscles and no rest. John complained of pain in his chest and shoulders, rapid heartbeat, and shortness of breath. The symptoms often occurred after light exertion such as walking up stairs and during times of emotional stress. In an exploration, John recalled a series of memories that led him back to the sensitizing events.

When John was fourteen years old, he decided to leave home. He could no longer tolerate his father's bad temper. As he was walking out the door, his father (who had a heart condition) told John that the upset caused by his leaving might cause another heart attack. John left with a tremendous feeling of guilt, but he knew he had to go. A week later he got word that his father did indeed have a serious heart attack.

John then recalled a memory of a time when he was twelve years old. His father was taking him to a factory to get a job. The factory owner refused to hire him until his thirteenth birthday because of child labor laws. John's father grabbed John's shoulder and in a fit of anger dragged him out of the factory. The next memory went back to a time when John was a young child, lying in his crib feeling lonely and unhappy. John began to cry, disturbing his father's nap. His father came in with an angry and "cold hearted" response. John recalled his fear and the crying and feeling short of breath.

In remembering the guilt he felt after his father's heart attack, the pain in his shoulder when his father had

169

grabbed him, and the shortness of breath when he was a baby, John could see how he had built his symptoms into his self-image. His father was such a threat to him that he began to focus stress on his own heart—unconsciously remembering the anxiety of his father's threat when he was leaving home as a boy. In a relaxed state, John could see that he was not to blame for his father's heart attack and that he needn't continue to fear his father's anger. This new adjustment in John's self-image resulted in a decrease in his heart rate. His other symptoms began to improve soon afterward.

This case is an excellent example of how emotional stresses can be linked to physical symptoms. Often we cannot trace a physical symptom back to a *single* event. In many cases, the circumstances where the tension first occurred may not be traumatic to us. After several *similar events* the mind will begin to generalize the tension, and it will grow stronger. When we are young, much of the tension goes unnoticed. The heart is strong and receives a healthy blood supply during youth. As we grow older, many of us may reach the stage of spasm in the coronary arteries as John did. A tremendous number of diseases are a culmination of a lifetime of stress on the blood vessels and the heart's circulatory system. When we are older, only a small stress might cause a serious symptom as our reserves become limited.

Imagine that each time you relax and release the day's tension you are allowing your natural healing abilities to keep your body healthy and in balance and preventing the accumulation of tensions that lead to diseases. *Every time* you adaptively deal with a stress situation, you prolong the strength of your heart and your vascular system. Oftentimes changes in lifestyle can serve to reduce severe stress.

Dorothy is a sixty-five-year-old woman who came in for treatment for symptoms of heart failure—she experienced fatigue, shortness of breath, and swollen ankles. Dorothy owned a small business that she ran alone; she was constantly under pressure. She started appropriate medication for her heart condition. We discussed that it was essential that she not exert herself. She mentioned that her business was taking all her time; and she dreaded going every morning, but she felt she *had to go*! In an exploration, she realized that she was always being driven by schedules and had never really learned how to relax. Her life history indicated that she was a perfect target for heart problems. She recalled how much pressure she had felt from her parents when she was young, and she was now putting that same pressure on herself.

After the exploration, Dorothy made a major change in her life. She had enough money that it wasn't necessary for her to work any longer, and she sold her business. She felt much better, and even the heart block that had been present on her electrocardiogram disappeared. She changed her self-image so that she could see herself relaxing and doing some of the things she'd put off for years. She began enjoying herself. These changes allowed her body to restore its natural balance. At sixty-five, she is now leading groups for people in her age group with similar stress problems.

Tumors and cancer

One of the most difficult problems facing medical science today is the treatment of cancer and tumors. These growths arise from the very cells of the patient with the disease. The normal rate of cell growth is changed, and the

171

normal destruction of abnormal cells is halted. This causes large masses of cells to form and appear as benign or malignant tumors.

Tumors and cancers represent imbalances in the processes that keep cells in order and functioning properly. In tumor and cancer cells, the usual restrictions on the production of new cells are not present, and/or the destruction of abnormal cells ceases. The appearance of a *few* abnormal cells is not unusual in the healthy individual. Each day we produce hundreds of thousands of new cells, a small percentage of which are abnormal and therefore destroyed by the body in a natural way. We may be producing potentially tumorous or cancerous cells each day! What, then, leads to imbalance in the usual regulating controls that break down abnormal cells? Is it possible that these unwanted cells may grow undetected by the body in the same way that we have observed unwanted physical symptoms, habits, and emotions to become firmly ingrained without conscious awareness? Is it possible that some tumors and cancers may appear as a result of a chain of sensitizing events that lead to imbalance in the mechanism of cell regulation? Though no firm conclusions are available at this point, patients with these problems are being treated with the new methods we've been discussing. Fear, sadness, and tension are believed by many to play a significant part in the development of these diseases. This may have profound consequences for the treatment and cure of cancer and tumors in the next few years.

Some physicians are now beginning to use the meditative state and imagination to treat tumors and cancer. Carl Simonton, a radiologist and radiation cancer treatment specialist, has had significant results using these tools.

Simonton's work teaches relaxation and uses imagination to build up the expectation of remission and health. The cultural attitude toward cancer is very negative—many people believe that a diagnosis of cancer means certain death. This is false. Simonton's work has shown that this attitude can be reversed in favor of more optimistic expectations. In his work, he asks his patients to visualize the cancer and then visualize the white blood cells destroying it. Each individual has unique images. There is evidence that these techniques precipitate remission of the cancer

DENISE

Denise came in for treatment of an ovarian cyst. She had been told by another physician that it was the size of a orange, and surgery was suggested. Denise had heard stories of spontaneous remission of abnormal masses and tumors, and she wanted to explore any other possibilities before agreeing to surgery.

In a deep state of relaxation, we asked her nonconscious mind why the cyst was present—what did it represent in her life? The memory that bubbled up from her nonconscious was a disagreement with her husband. She deeply wanted a child and her husband didn't. He felt that it was the wrong time to have a child.

Out of her strong desire for a child, it seems her body had created a growth on her ovary. While relaxed, Denise could focus on the sensations in her ovaries. (Remember that in the relaxed state, attention can be acutely focused.) She described the cyst as feeling like a fluid-filled bag.

After the exploration, Denise was surprised that her body could so strongly respond to her psychological desires. Once this awareness had been brought to her conscious

attention and she understood it, her body no longer
needed to respond maladaptively. In one week the cyst had
disappeared!

JACK

Jack came in frightened by his physical symptoms. He had
a tumor in his prostate gland that had metastasized, and
there were suspicious nodules in his chest. Jack had seen
several doctors and was facing a biopsy, anticancer drugs,
and therapy. Treatment with female hormones was
suggested by one doctor. Jack began to panic at this point;
he was losing sleep; he had no appetite, and began to lose
weight. He associated all his symptoms with cancer.

In an exploration, Jack wanted to discover the source of his
fear. He realized that he had been strongly influenced by
his doctors and the symptoms of other people. He began
practicing relaxation processes several times a day and vis-
ualized the nodules and tumor shrinking. Along with this,
he began hormone treatment; in several weeks the tumor
was smaller, and the nodules in his chest had disappeared!
Most important, he felt confident, relaxed, and responsible
for his own health.

Jack's case is a good example of the importance of motivation in healing. He was willing to take the responsibility for
his cancer and work daily on his own to change his fear to
positive expectations. He feels that the hormones were
helpful but that his own efforts were central to his remission.

Although actual clinical research on this approach to
cancer is just beginning, the idea that cancer is related to
stress and self-image is not new. In 1959 Eugene Pender-
gass, ex-president of the American Cancer Society, stated:

> ... I personally observed cancer patients who have un-
> dergone successful treatment and were living and well for
> years. Then an emotional stress such as the death of a son
> in World War II, the infidelity of a daughter-in-law or the
> burden of long unemployment seems to have been the pre-
> cipitating factor in the reactivation of their disease which
> resulted in death. ... There is solid evidence that the
> course of disease in general is affected by emotional dis-
> tress ... thus we as doctors may begin to emphasize treat-
> ment of the patient as a whole as well as the disease from
> which the patient is suffering.[1]

Little is known about what actual percentage of
exacerbations or remissions are related in a cause-and-
effect way to changes in self-image. What we do know for
sure is that the use of these tools changes the mental outlook of the patient; and what's more, even in the case of
those who do eventually die from the tumor, their last
weeks and days are enjoyable, the quality of their life is
improved. Future research will no doubt elucidate more
fully the role of the mind in cancer.

Dentistry

Most of us expect that when we visit the dentist we are
sure to experience some pain and discomfort. Again, as we
have observed many times, the expectation of pain and the
accompanying fear may indeed produce the pain! As we
now know, it doesn't have to be that way. Many dentists are

[1] Eugene Pendergrass, quoted by Kenneth Pelletier, *Mind as Healer,
Mind as Slayer* (New York: Delta, 1977), p. 148.

trained in techniques of deep relaxation. They often will suggest to the patient that he or she imagine the teeth as little blocks of wood and the gums as frozen, or they may suggest other images associated with numbness.

In a state of deep relaxation, an oral surgeon performing a complicated tooth extraction may suggest to the patient that he or she keep the area around the tooth dry and clear of blood. Following the extraction, when blood is needed in the area to form a clot, the patient might then be asked to imagine that blood is filling the socket where the tooth has been extracted. The control of the patient might seem startling; the blood will often flow until the tooth socket is filled exactly to the brim and then stop!

AL

Al complained of a serious toothache and had been taking pain relievers for several weeks. He knew that it was inevitable that he would have to go to the dentist, but his lifelong nervousness about the dentist's office kept him procrastinating. He began to build up so much anxiety over his toothache that he came in for an exploration to find the source of his fear, which he knew was out of proportion. In the exploration Al recalled a situation when he was young. He was sitting in the dentist's chair waiting for an examination while in the next room he could hear the buzzing of the drill and a young girl crying in pain. His nonconscious mind remembered the fear associated with the sounds of the dentist's office, and now that he was facing a tooth extraction the anxiety was reevoked to the point that Al's daily behavior became maladaptive. Al worked on his self-image in relation to his fear of the dentist's office and in a couple of weeks had his tooth extracted. He used no anesthesia; instead he used deep relaxation, felt no pain, and had no further complications.

Several weeks later Al came in for another visit. He was happy about overcoming his fear of dentists, but something more exciting had occurred since his tooth extraction. For months he'd been trying to quit smoking with no success. After his visit to the dentist, he decided to try again. To his surprise this time was remarkably easy—he hadn't smoked for weeks and had no desire to start again. The usual frustration and anxiety over not having a cigarette did not occur. Al had come to the office this time for an explanation!

Here we see an example of the principle of *generalization* that we discussed earlier. For the first time Al had learned that he could be in control of his own responses. The realization that he no longer had to live with his fear of the dentist's office and that he could even have dental work done without novocain or other anesthesia had a profound effect on him. He had learned new tools that allowed him to be responsible for and in control of his own healing processes rather than being the victim of old, unconscious patterns. This insight generalized to Al's smoking problem. He now could see that *he* could be in control of the problem if he decided to do so.

This is a common occurrence with these processes where the patient plays a significant role in the treatment and cure of a problem. Once a specific symptom, emotion, or habit pattern is resolved, the tools can be generalized to other areas. It's not surprising that many people report an overall increase in the quality of their lives after having recovered their natural tools!

A panacea?

I believe that just about all human beings can benefit from the understanding and awareness that is possible through techniques of self-discovery, such as the selective awareness exploration. Yet I do not believe that all diseases can be cured in this manner. Indeed, in my experience not even all those diseases produced through psychosomatic mechanisms have yielded fully to these techniques.

Many factors come into play, and together they determine how successful we will be in any given case. I will mention a few of these factors.

First of all, the individual must be willing and motivated. You might ask yourself, "How could a person not be motivated to get rid of a maladaptive symptom, habit pattern, or emotion?" You can answer this for yourself by asking several people you know who smoke whether they would be interested in putting effort into breaking their habit. Ask those who drink alcohol on a regular basis if they want to quit. Although some might be interested, many are not. The exploration would fail in their cases. Every once in a while, some parent of an unruly teen-ager comes into my office and demands that I "reprogram" the youngster. As I look into the glaring eyes of my prospective patient, I know right away that it would be an utter failure. Willingness and motivation are necessary to produce the cooperation required to begin to entice the nonconscious mind to reveal its secrets and to allow the initiation of a new pattern.

A person must permit him/herself to relax. Some people "don't see the value of relaxation" and are not interested in trying it. Some become bored during the process of relaxing the body and thus never achieve even the lighter levels of relaxation. Without this relaxation, we cannot make the proper contact with the nonconscious mind, the autonomic nervous system, or the deeper emotions—thus severely limiting the potential of this technique.

Still other people find it very difficult to detect emotions within themselves. Since this approach depends to some degree upon people's allowing themselves to feel what is happening within, I sometimes suggest that preliminary work in relaxation and self-awareness precede the actual exploration. Once the person feels more comfortable in experiencing and expressing emotion, the exploration is much more effective.

Some people want magic. They think that they will sit down and close their eyes and awake to find themselves healed in an hour. They do not intend to do any work; and although the exploration is based on relaxation, quite a bit of physical, emotional, and mental work often takes place when powerful memories emerge. The lazy do not fare well.

Some people can produce good visual images, some people produce good auditory imagery, and still others excel at bodily imagery and movement. Any or all of these kinds of imagery can serve to put us in contact with the nonconscious during the exploration.

After a stroke or brain damage or in senility, the effect of these approaches is markedly decreased. Similarly, in retarded individuals there is often insufficient capacity to accomplish very much through these techniques. Success is most likely in the most intelligent.

Sometimes an individual comes in for treatment too late. In our culture we tend to be very crisis oriented—we will endure stress, tension, and very disturbing symptoms for a long time, then finally show up for help when things are about to collapse completely. An ulcer patient can expect very good healing early in the disease; yet after many years of recurrent bleeding, scar tissue will have formed around the ulcer. Although it would be possible for him or her to change the self-image, behavior, and response to stressful situations, the scar tissue might still be so thick that healing cannot take place; and the ulcer will remain. The man with the gangrene of the toes could not have cured the disease had they been amputated prior to his coming to me. He might have learned the behavioral change, but the physical change would have been impossible. An organ of the body that has been damaged beyond repair through psychosomatic mechanisms is just as irreparable as an organ that has been damaged beyond repair by physical trauma.

In most cases, it is necessary for an individual to spend several days or several weeks rewriting maladaptive patterns and projecting a desirable self-image in order to completely reverse an established pattern. Negative patterns are very well learned by the mind, and it takes time to learn a new response. Many people fail to put in sufficient time, and although the exploration might have made it very clear what the pattern was and how it could be changed, a lack of motivation can nullify this. A can of paint still requires a painter to put it on the wall. Frequent use of the tapes with the attendant access to the deeper levels of mind and body generally leads to much greater improvement.

No, this is not a panacea. In spite of all the remarkable things that have been observed, we must keep in mind that these approaches are still in their infancy. I suspect that as more and more is learned about the relationship of mind and body and as more techniques become available for increasing mind–body harmony an even greater percentage of successes will be possible.[2]

---

[2]See Appendix. Several approaches to facilitating the healing process can be found on the following tapes: "Selective Awareness Introductory Tape" (#10) and "Healing Journey Tape" (#16).

III
You and medical science— the implications

The mice in council

For many years the mice had been living in constant dread of their enemy, the cat. It was decided to call a meeting to determine the best means of handling the situation. Many plans were discussed and rejected.

At last a young mouse got up. "I propose," said he, looking very important, "that a bell be hung around the cat's neck. Then whenever the cat approaches, we always shall have notice of her presence, and so be able to escape.

The young mouse sat down amidst tremendous applause. The suggestion was put to a motion and passed almost unanimously.

But just then an old mouse, who had sat silent all the while, rose to his feet and said: "My friends, it takes a young mouse to think of a plan so ingenious and yet so simple. With a bell about the cat's neck to warn us we shall all be safe. I have but one brief

*question to put to the supporters of the plan—which one of you is
going to bell the cat?"*

APPLICATION: It is one thing to propose, another to exe-
cute.

The ants and the pen

*An ant one day strayed across a piece of paper and saw a pen
writing in fine, black strokes.*

*"How wonderful this is!" said the ant. "This remarkable
thing, with a life of its own, makes squiggles on this beautiful
surface, to such an extent and with such energy that it is equal to
the efforts of all the ants in the world. And the squiggles which it
makes! These resemble ants—not one, but millions, all run together."*

*He repeated his ideas to another ant, who was equally in-
terested. He praised the powers of observation and reflection of the
first ant.*

*But another ant said: "Profiting, it must be admitted, by your
efforts, I have observed this strange object. But, I have determined
that it is not the master of this work. You fail to notice that this pen
is attached to certain other objects, which surround it and drive it
on its way. These should be considered as the moving factor and
given the credit." Thus were fingers discovered by the ants.*

*But another ant, after a long time, climbed over the fingers
and realised that they comprised a hand, which he thoroughly
explored after the manner of ants, by scrambling all over it.*

*He returned to his fellows: "Ants!" he cried, "I have news of
importance for you. Those smaller objects are a part of a large one.
It is this which gives motion to them."*

But then it was discovered that the hand was attached to an arm and the arm to a body, and that there were two hands, and that there were feet which did no writing.

The investigation continued. Of the mechanics of writing the ants have a fair idea. Of the meaning and intension of the writing, and how it is ultimately controlled, they will not find out by their customary method of investigation.

Introduction to part III

Now that you've seen how the processes of relaxation and imagination work to restore health and balance, we'll begin to focus more directly on *you!* In Chapter 12 we talk about the essential ingredient that allows these processes to work for each individual. We also answer some questions you might have about using these tools for yourself. Then we look at some simple, practical applications of the processes that you can use in your everyday life in Chapter 13.

Chapters 14 and 15 discuss some of the differences between traditional medical science and the broader view of medicine (often called *holistic* medicine) that we've been exploring. We look at the powerful role of the doctor in our culture and how we need to reevaluate our old notions of effective health care.

Now would be a good opportunity to reflect on the medical care you've had in the last few years. Are you satisfied with it? Do you want more? What would you like to do to improve your health and the health of your family? If you could make recommendations on how to improve health care in our culture, what would you suggest?

12

How about you?

The boy and the nettle

A boy playing in the fields one day was stung in the hand by a nettle. Running home to his mother he cried: "See what the nasty weed did to me. I barely touched it when it buried its prickers in my hand."

"It was because you touched it lightly," replied the boy's mother, "that it stung you. The next time, dear son, that you play with a nettle, grasp it tightly, and it will do you no harm."

APPLICATION: Do boldly what you do at all.

Is this for you?

Many people are now just beginning to discover that their natural healing abilities can improve their health and

187

the quality of their lives. The main factor in the success of the approaches presented in this book is the *motivation* of each individual—the desire and willingness to "make it work" or better still, to "let it happen"! Some of us may find it difficult to overcome old cultural notions about medicine and healing. Our cherished beliefs that we are helpless victims of germs, microorganisms, and the crippling diseases of age are being challenged. In order for us to accept a new point of view, we may need to readjust our self-images. The key to doing this lies in accepting ourselves the way we are with the healing abilities that we all possess—even though we may never have consciously used them before.

We must face the fear of the new and the unknown. With respect to new frontiers in medicine, one may be like a bird who has been caged for years and is then set free, only to fight one's way back into the cage—not knowing what to do with the freedom. It takes strength to be a pioneer.

With freedom comes increased responsibility. Responsibility means that you are willing to handle your physical symptoms directly, not helplessly hoping that someone will tell you how to make them go away. Such notions as "I can't help myself" must be replaced by "I can" or "I am willing." Responsibility also means that the goals you choose must be potentially possible and reasonable, not unrealistic, frivolous wishful thinking. You must be willing to give your self-image a chance to adjust itself; the process will be gradual. You've read all the case histories in the last chapter; each of these people was patient and willing to make responsible changes in their lives—and they were successful! A responsible attitude would be like "losing" your temper and being willing to "find" it again.

All individuals must ask themselves if they are willing to take on this responsibility. For many of us, it's not an easy task. Each time we gain more power and freedom, we have to be willing to trust ourselves, to have the confidence to make the right decisions and carry them through, to forgive ourselves when we make mistakes, and to move on to new challenges. There's a tremendous amount of power and satisfaction in self-control. We all know what that experience is like—remember the pride and excitement you experienced when you first rode a bicycle, when you were young and first bought a present for someone you cared about all by yourself, when you first drove a car, when you first moved away from home and were on your own, your first job or your first day of college, and all those other important "firsts" that gave you new freedom and responsibility? Do you recall the satisfaction that made it all worthwhile?

Some people are unable to give up their physical symptoms. These people use a symptom as an excuse, a scapegoat on which to blame their troubles. The woman who's had arthritis for thirty years needs to be served and waited on; every time she is called upon to do something for herself, she uses her arthritis as an excuse. Without her symptoms, she would have to find another way to escape the responsibilities of life. For people in similar situations, giving up a recurrent symptom would create severe turbulence. Another example is the man who came in to be treated for migraine headaches. Every time he began to have a severe headache, he would call his son and daughter who lived in nearby towns to come and care for him. He learned relaxation tools and was able to control his headaches. But the root of his problem was much deeper. When he no longer had migraine headaches, his son and daughter stopped visiting, since he was no longer in distress. He could not cope with the feelings of loneliness and was unwilling to explore why his children didn't enjoy visiting him. His headaches had given him a means by which to maintain contact with them. Even though he had learned the tools to alleviate his headaches, he was unwilling to use them and face the underlying problems. So he stopped practicing his relaxation procedures, his headaches returned, and his family began to visit him again. These processes are not for everyone. They are only for those who are motivated to be healthy and take the responsibility that comes along with that.

This factor has always been an important one when autogenic methods of healing are employed. One well-known phenomenon in hypnosis demonstrates that fact. We know that it is often quite easy when working with a good hypnotic subject to give a suggestion that a habit—such as smoking or overeating—or a symptom—like a headache or stomach-ache—will vanish. The suggestion works dramatically—for a few days or weeks—but the problem returns. This is because a symptom is often not a disconnected fragment but an integral part of our lives, woven into the fabric of our self-image. An awareness of this fact and the acceptance of the challenge to change on a deeper level are often prerequisites for full healing.

Experiments done in the laboratory haven't as yet been able to show the extent to which we can produce physical, emotional, and mental changes in ourselves. As we have discovered, motivation is a key factor. In laboratory studies, the motivation of the subject is often limited to a small financial reward and pleasing the experimenter with good results. It would be more meaningful to test the strength of these processes with subjects who stand to significantly improve their health and the quality of their lives. For example, suppose a research team were testing the ability of a subject group to control their blood pressure. The usual procedure would be to choose a random experimental group from a hypertensive clinic population. If, however, one were to choose a group of patients who believed that they could truly learn to help themselves and who were motivated to put forth effort and assume the responsibility, we might expect the percentage of those successful in producing a positive change to be much higher. Perhaps the future will give us more evidence to back this up.

Often in our culture we have the habit of looking for the flaws in new systems. If we find one, we often call the whole system useless and discard it. We must be aware of the tendency to throw out the baby with the bath water. The approaches to self-healing discussed here do not as yet form a comprehensive system or theory, nor are they always successful. We are dealing with the uniqueness of each individual case. Yet a growing number of people are finding help, relief, and a new perspective on life through these techniques. Sometimes the change is subtle, sometimes dramatic. The goal of this book is to give you some new information so that *you* can choose what is appropriate in your life.

How do you know for sure?

The cases presented so far can give you an idea of how health and balance can be restored through the use of natural relaxation and imagination. They are not to be used to compare with your own physical symptoms. Each of you is unique, and therefore each case will be different. We can, however, offer you some general comments about using these processes for yourself. We've anticipated some of the questions you might have.

What is the difference between relaxation and deep relaxation?

In this book we have used the term *relaxation* in two contexts. During the practice of meditation, autogenic training, self-hypnosis, or in the selective awareness state—one experiences *deep relaxation*. This is characterized by stillness, slow breathing, and a minimum of analytical thoughts. This is the most effective state for producing imagery, interacting with that imagery, increasing self-awareness, and for communicating with the deeper levels of the mind. This deep relaxation alone, or in combination with other techniques, helps facilitate a return to physiological balance. One rarely uses this specialized state for more than five to fifteen minutes at a time.

Relaxation differs from *deep relaxation* in that during *relaxation*, one is alert to outside stimuli, may be in vigorous motion, and may perform analytical tasks; yet there is a sense of calm and a lack of anxiety and static tension. Muscles alternately contract and relax, and the mind functions creatively, free from the mental tension that would bind it to fear-producing images. Except in times of immediate physical danger, *relaxation* represents the normal, balanced, physiological state of the mind and body.

What if I find it difficult to reach a state of deep relaxation?

The ability to experience a deep state of relaxation is available to everyone. Through childhood, in school, and in your jobs you may have had little opportunity to teach your body and your mind how to relax. Biofeedback, meditation, autogenic training, and yoga can help you to learn this process. If you decide to use the tapes described at the end of this book, you will find that you can easily reach the relaxed state in from three to ten sessions. The next step is learning to *produce* the state of deep relaxation without tape or guide so you can call on it in any situation you choose. Some people may learn this in a few days; other may take weeks or months. Don't push yourself. Remember, relaxation is a natural healing state. If you've spent your whole life with pressures and time schedules, it may take you a little time.

Tension, anxiety, and nervousness are symptoms; and the longer we've had them, the deeper they penetrate into the heart of our self-image. Through them, the mind tries to help avoid shocks and surprises. It will take time for the mind of an intelligent being to learn to trust the state of relaxation—to know on a deep level that it is okay to "let go."

Once you are familiar with the pathway from tension to relaxation, you will find that you automatically relax at times you previously tensed up and that you can consciously choose to use it in a stressful situation, during an argument, or when you're beginning to feel unbalanced. You will develop the proper timing and correct response to keep youself in balance just as you learned to ride a bike effortlessly. Every moment spent learning these processes will be repaid many times over.

Suppose I become uncomfortable when I try to relax?

Sometimes people tell me after their first practice session in deep relaxation: "I've been trying to relax, but it seems as though my muscles feel *more* tense." In most cases, this is a good sign. Many people carry maladaptive tension around with them for years and lose their sensitivity to it. Make a tight fist and maintain it for five to ten minutes. At first it hurts; then it gets numb. When you relax it again, the pain briefly starts up. When you first begin to relax and focus on your internal awareness, the inner tension, worry, and concern may seem more noticeable than before. That's all right. It takes time for the mind to give up old patterns, and the first step is to let yourself discover them. Getting through this stage requires a little patience and willingness to become more sensitive to the signals from your body. Then you can begin to control the levels of tension. It's much like learning to ride a bicycle. In the beginning, you are clumsy and awkward, trying to coordinate your arms and legs and maintain your balance all at once. If you avoid the clumsy phase by not getting on the bicycle, you never learn. If you are motivated to learn to ride, you will keep working at it and reach a point where you can ride effortlessly and relaxedly—you maintain your balance automatically and *naturally*. So it is with relaxation. Once learned it becomes a natural tool that you can call on at any time.

You may imagine that learning these processes is much like planting a seed in a garden. When you first plant the seed, you must carefully and gently water it each day, even though there are no visible signs of sprouting. If you are patient and continue to care for it, soon you will see a small shoot that may later grow into a beautiful flower. When you are learning to relax, you may find it a bit difficult at first and not notice any real change. But the seed is growing underground, and soon it will sprout to let you know that your efforts are being rewarded!

Once you learn to master the state of relaxation, you will still be able to become angry, to experience fear in front of a large group of people; you even will still have the potential of developing an ulcer; but now you will also have the choice of relaxing and choosing a different pathway. The state of relaxation is a natural one that allows you more freedom to choose the lifestyle you prefer and to live more efficiently and enjoyably. It never forces you to do anything.

If you find yourself saying, "I can't," look more closely and see if you really mean "I won't!" The ingrained maladaptive patterns in your mind may be resisting; if you stay with it, you can be sure of your reward.

Can I use these processes if I'm already taking prescribed medication and am under a doctor's care?

Yes. Many people have found that when they begin to learn relaxation processes, the natural healing mechanisms of the body begin doing the work that the medication was doing. Tell your doctor that you plan to learn these processes. Perhaps suggest that he or she read portions of this book that you think are particularly relevant to you. Most doctors will be happy to hear about this information. Let your doctor know if you'll be practicing with some of the tapes discussed at the end of the book. With his knowledge of the body he may be able to suggest some effective ways of using your imagery. You and your doctor may notice that your general health and well-being begin to improve when you learn these processes, at which time your doctor may want to gradually withdraw part or all of the medication and let your body resume the job of maintaining its own balance. People with hypertension, for example, often can learn to control their blood pressure on their own and no longer need medication. Similarly, after learning these techniques, patients have been able to reduce or eliminate—under a physician's supervision—the use of such medications as tranquilizers, cortisone, muscle relaxants, hormones, pain pills, antispasmodics, and antihistamines. Can you imagine your body taking over the job that a medicine has been doing for you?

How can I get started in learning more about these tools?

The number of physicians, therapists, counselors, and clergymen who are using relaxation tools is growing rapidly. The actual techniques, however, are *not* the most important aspects of this new view of medical science. Your attitude about your ability to be in control of your own health and well-being is *central*. You may decide to use the prepared tapes, autogenic training, meditation, yoga, or biofeedback techniques—all are excellent introductions to the deeply relaxed state.

If you're interested in exploring the possibilities that we've been discussing, don't wait until something goes wrong with your mental or physical health—start today. Don't fall prey to the old crisis orientation that has plagued the practitioners of traditional medicine. An ounce of prevention is still worth a pound of cure.

Take your time. Begin to notice your own patterns, the familiar symptoms that you experience in your daily life; and observe how you respond in stressful, tense situations. This will allow you to clarify your own goals in using these processes. Talk to your doctor and other health professionals in your community. You will find people in your area who are doing similar work. Maybe you know some doctors in your community who would be interested in expanding their medical practice to include these tools. They might wish to read this book or the other books and articles listed in the bibliography.[1] Remember, you're in charge now, if you want to be.

Do I have to believe in these processes for them to work?

Remember that the conscious mind does not work in the same way as does the nonconscious. At this point, you may not be able to clearly imagine how your nonconscious mind actually stores all the experiences of your life. If you're inclined to see if these tools work for you—try them. Ask yourself the question, "Exactly what is it that I don't believe? What parts are difficult for me to accept?" Use the bibliography in the back, ask your doctor, talk to your friends, and explore the answer for yourself. Trust yourself to know what's right for you. Be aware that asking such questions as, "Can I dare to believe that I can be successful at this?" may be an old, maladaptive pattern for you; do you ever give yourself excuses to keep yourself from starting new projects?

Are these processes safe for me to use?

Yes. These processes are safer than taking aspirin. They allow you to rediscover your *natural* abilities. You may discover that you experience changes in your mental and emotional outlook; some of them may be a bit unsettling, and some may open the door for you to experience new areas of your life. In order to experience more health

---

[1]*Selective Awareness* (3rd ed.) and the "Selective Awareness Introductory Tape" (10) provide a good way to get started in learning more about these processes.

and well-being in your life, you first must clear out some of the cobwebs that have been keeping you stuck in old patterns.

If I can recall no incidents from my childhood that seem "traumatic," might there still be a need to explore my early years?

Events that cause the nonconscious mind to create physical symptoms are not necessarily terrifying or confusing to the adult mind. However, when they occurred, they may have caused tension and fear to be associated with a specific area of the body that the mind interpreted as a threat to survival.

Imagine a baby soon after birth. At first she simply lies in her crib. After a few weeks she is able to follow things around the room with her eyes. She can wiggle her arms and legs and may smile at her mother and father but has few other ways to respond to the environment. One day she discovers that she can move things with her hands! When the discovery is noticed by her parents, she begins to get toys—rattles, blocks, furry stuffed animals. She soon begins using her hands to put everything in her mouth. She realizes that she can play games with her new toys— she can throw them out of the crib, and Mom and Dad will happily return them time after time!

As she grows older, she learns to stand in the playpen. It is filled with toys, and she is allowed to touch everything within reach. She is in control of her little environment and continues to use her hands to explore. Soon she is allowed out of the playpen and begins to crawl around on the floor. She is excited about all the new places to explore.

For months she has been noticing the shiny glass dish on the coffee table; now she finally has the chance to play with it. As she crawls over to the coffee table and begins to reach for her new toy, she suddenly hears "NO!" and her mother swiftly picks her up and puts her back in the playpen. Never before has she been restricted from touching anything within reach. The next times she is crawling on the floor, she again reaches for the shiny object. She takes it in her hands and again hears a loud "NO!" and the dish is taken away. She begins to cry in frustration and confusion. The next time she reaches for the dish, she gets a slap on the hand; and the dish is moved to a higher shelf, completely out of her reach, leaving her discouraged and unhappy.

We all know that circumstances such as these occur all the time during childhood. No serious harm is done—the child must learn which objects she can play with and which ones are forbidden or dangerous. But how does it look through the eyes of the child? When she is punished, her attention is completely focused on that moment. She is not aware of the wonderful times she has when her parents take her out in the stroller; she doesn't think about how much her parents love her. She doesn't have friends to whom she can go to discuss her confusion and pain. She only has the shiny glass object in her mind. She wants to explore and play, and when she is interrupted, her world is momentarily shattered. As we know, children can cry one moment and laugh the next. But if this experience occurs time after time after time, the child may experience the beginning of a maladaptive way of looking at life. This is what the child's mind might record:

> The World is a beautiful place, and I can explore with my hands, There are many things to touch with my hands,

but some things are dangerous. If I touch them, I will be yelled at and spanked. What's worse, there's no way to tell beforehand whether or not I can touch a particular thing. It seems that the things that are new, unusual, shiny, and beautiful are the most dangerous to touch.

Of course, as children grow up they begin to understand why certain behavior is dangerous; but if the early experiences were confusing and highly charged with emotion, the basic message above may remain in the deeper levels of the mind. If the child grows up in an environment where there are numerous rules and forbidden actions she does not comprehend, this message may be permanently built into her self-image. Is it any wonder that many of us grow up lacking confidence, afraid to "reach out" to new challenges, to our friends and the people we love? Is it any wonder that it's difficult to "touch" new and beautiful experiences, to leave the secure, routine, everyday patterns of life and try something completely new? Is it any wonder that so many of us are at times "caught in a rut" and do nothing about it for fear of "getting our hands slapped"? How often do we complain about the way we live and see how beautiful things are elsewhere—outside of our "playpen"?

We can see that not only "traumatic" events can set up negative self-images. Often the day-to-day frustrations of childhood and all of life can be the roots of our problems. Human children are often punished for "social" misdeeds that don't make sense to our basic nature. The mind sees being punished as threatening and looks for some way to escape. The escape may be to build a self-image that says "I'm too shy" or "I have no confidence." People with these

aspects to their self-image may escape the pain and fear of
failure by never venturing out. They would rather live
with the same old routine every day than take risks. The
exploration is a way of tracing events through our lives,
keeping our minds relaxed so we will not "run away."

Think about some of the things you'd really like to do
but somehow haven't been able to get around to. Would
you like to leave your job and get a better one? To travel?
Would you like to begin a new hobby or move to another
neighborhood? Another city, state, or country? Is there
some person or group of people you'd like to get better
acquainted with but somehow haven't had the courage to
approach? Is there a habit you'd like to break but haven't
been able to overcome?

We all may have some of these characteristics to a
greater or lesser degree. Frustrations and discourage-
ments have been collected over the years by the mind,
which may have caused negative aspects to be built into the
self-image. These aspects may constantly be there like a
nagging voice in the back of the head telling us that we're
not successful, questioning our goals, causing us to slow
down and pause and doubt when we want to move forward. With the slightest falter, the least pause, the smallest
imperfection, that voice begins to convince us that we are
going to fail. We begin to doubt ourselves and feel uncer-
tain, which causes tension—tension that often causes
further mistakes. And the cycle continues.

With the processes of relaxation we can tap more of
the potential of the human mind; we can use the storage
capacity of the nonconscious mind as a resource to help us
solve problems, be more creative, and bring more satisfaction into our lives.

SAM

Whenever Sam had to travel any distance in the back seat of a car, he became car-sick. Curiously he had no difficulty when he rode in the front seat. During an exploration Sam discovered a memory dating back to his first year of life.

Sam's mother had to be taken to the hospital for surgery. Sam had been with his mother day and night since birth, and he was extremely frightened. During her hospital stay, Sam was to live with his aunt and uncle. As his uncle was driving away from the hospital, his aunt tried to calm Sam by playing games with him in the back seat. But he could not seem to stop crying. As he saw the hospital fade away into the distance out the back window of the car, Sam felt lonely, afraid, and anxious.

This experience was recalled by his nonconscious mind every time he got into the back seat of a car. His mind was reminding him that back seats were threatening and dangerous to him—that they caused him tremendous pain and anxiety. The emotional tension and anxiety were converted into dizziness, nausea, and feelings of being trapped. These symptoms served the purpose of getting Sam to move out of the back seat.

Once this memory became conscious with all the emotions that were present, Sam could understand how his mind had created the physical symptoms resulting from the fear he experienced when he was away from his mother. He relived the memory with the understanding that his mother would be gone only a few days and that he would be taken care of by his aunt and uncle. He also relived other memories of being in the back seat of a car rewriting them according to the new, more adaptive pattern to rid himself of his maladaptive response. With this adjustment of his self-image the pattern faded rapidly, and Sam could comfortably ride in back seats.

Prior to his exploration, Sam had, on many occasions, recalled part of this memory but never had any strong feelings about it. When he relived it in the deeply relaxed state, however, all the original emotions came to the surface, and Sam wept bitterly during his first time through the memory. As he rewrote it the second time, he was calm.

It is very common during an exploration to discover powerful emotions in a memory that has always seemed bland. The nonconscious does this to "protect" us from these emotions; yet until we relax enough to release these stored up feelings, they can continue to be the driving force behind our most troublesome patterns.

Is it always necessary to go back to childhood to resolve a maladaptive pattern?

No! Sometimes an exploration that extends back only a few years will do the job. However, there's no way to know beforehand how far back the nonconscious will guide us. Often people who are certain their pattern will trace back only a short way end up going back to the very earliest period of their lives; thus it's best not to preprogram the experience—just trust the nonconscious, and see where it leads.

Generally speaking, the more severe or illogical a maladaptive pattern, the more likely it is to date back to very early years or to a very traumatic event in adult life; since these are the times when judgment is poorest, and when poor solutions (escape patterns) are selected.

We have seen how the ability to focus awareness gives us more control over our minds and bodies. We have seen how it is possible to control everyday tension and stress and to prevent them from becoming maladaptive. So let's begin to look at some of the "little things" in life that happen every day so we can begin to put these notions into practice now. You can see for yourself whether or not they work for you.

Have you ever accidentally hit your thumb with a hammer and yelled at the hammer? Or shut your finger in a car door and sworn at the door? Or lost your car keys and stomped around angrily tossing coats on the floor and rummaging through drawers? Have you ever been angry at a traffic light for turning red when you're late for an appointment? "How could I have been so stupid?" or "What an idiot I am"? Do you remember how you felt at those times?

These common situations can all create maladaptive tension in the body; and you may notice that the tension can last for hours, changing your whole perspective on the day ("I got up on the wrong side of the bed this morning, burned breakfast, was late to work, and it's been that way all day!"). Carrying maladaptive tension around during the day makes it difficult to feel satisfied and fulfilled in life. We all know people who haven't had a "really good day" in months. It is possible to eliminate these unnecessary responses in your life. Think of some specific situations in your life where you noticed unwanted tension. How did you feel? Now imagine how you might feel if you were free of that tension.

As we've seen, tension often builds up and becomes associated with a specific area of the body, which causes physical symptoms. By just being *aware* of the importance of releasing maladaptive tension, you may begin to notice changes in your life. Instead of hearing yourself say, "This whole day's been a waste; it started out all wrong when I dented the bumper of my car, and I couldn't think of anything else all day!", you might find yourself saying, "This morning I was really upset about denting the bumper for a while, but then I decided the tension was not helping me; so I chose to relax, and the rest of the day is going fine." The choice of relaxing gives your mind a chance to release the tension of the early morning situation so that you don't carry it with you into the rest of your day and into the evening.

Many people carry their maladaptive tensions further and may spend a week or more "crying the blues," telling everyone they run into about their terrible misfortune. Many of us have this nonconscious mechanism to enlist attention from others, but few realize that this can actually delay healing. How many times have you heard someone say, "I really wrecked (busted, destroyed, ruined, smashed, crushed) my foot yesterday!" It might be more reasonable to say, "Oh, yes, I bruised my toe yesterday, but it's nothing significant. In fact, it seems to be getting better already."

People like to dramatize their problems. It gives them something to talk about. We all know that bad news travels faster than good news. Have you ever noticed how much people enjoy telling others about their misfortunes? In a group, there is often a little skirmish after each story as the others vie for the right to tell their bummer first. The nonconscious may figure that if you're enjoying talking about your problem, it must be valuable or pleasurable to you in some way; so, in order to give you more happiness, it may actually retard the healing process or cause you to have other problems!

Tension and fear are the usual responses to an injury. The person who gets a shock while fixing a lamp usually jerks his or her hand away far out of proportion to the jolt itself, as does the person who inadvertently steps on a tack. This is a nonconscious response that is highly adaptive to protect the organism. These responses may become maladaptive if dramatized. Suppose a pianist cuts her hand while slicing an onion. She imagines, "Oh, no! If this is still sore on Suday, I'll give a poor performance at the recital and lose my scholarship!" She puts an image in her mind of herself still suffering from the cut on Sunday, which may *cause* her nonconscious mind to slow the healing process *and bring about the very thing she fears*. Whether the imagined consequences are realistic or not, it is maladaptive to create unnecessary tension and anxiety.

A dentist in California who is now using relaxation tools with his patients has clearly demonstrated the effect of belief and suggestion on the apparent healing rate. He carried out an experiment in his office in which patients who had had wisdom teeth extracted were divided into three groups. Those in the first group were given a list of postoperative instructions and a prescription for an analgesic. The instructions informed them of what should be done in the case of bleeding, swelling, or pain. Those in the second group were given the suggestion—without inducing the state of relaxation—that they would be fine and that they should call the office if they had any questions. (The semantics for this group were carefully chosen; patients were told to call the office if they had *questions*—not *problems*.) Patients in the third group were placed in a state of deep relaxation, and the suggestion was given that pain, bleeding, and swelling *would not be experienced* after the extraction.

Pain — None · Mild · Moderate · Severe
Swelling — None · Mild · Moderate · Severe
Bleeding — None · Mild · Moderate · Severe

Post-Op Instructions and Prescription

	Pain None	Mild	Moderate	Severe	Swelling None	Mild	Moderate	Severe	Bleeding None	Mild	Moderate	Severe
1 Routine extraction	////	/			卌				////			
2 Tissue impaction		//				//			///	/		
3 Surgical extraction			/	/		/	//		/		///	
4 Partial bony impaction			/	////*			//	//			//	
5 Bony impaction				//				//				/

Waking Suggestion

	Pain None	Mild	Moderate	Severe	Swelling None	Mild	Moderate	Severe	Bleeding None	Mild	Moderate	Severe
1 Routine extraction	卌 //	/			卌 ///	/			卌 ///	//		
2 Tissue impaction	/	/			/	/			/	/		
3 Surgical extraction			/	/*	/		//		//		/	
4 Partial bony impaction	/											
5 Bony impaction					//							

Suggestion and Deep Relaxation

	Pain None	Mild	Moderate	Severe	Swelling None	Mild	Moderate	Severe	Bleeding None	Mild	Moderate	Severe
1 Routine extraction	卌 /				卌 /				卌 /			
2 Tissue impaction	//				//	/			/			
3 Surgical extraction	//				//	/			///	/		
4 Partial bony impaction		/				/			/			
5 Bony impaction		//			//	//			////			

*Dry socket

Figure 12-1

Patients were seen one week after extraction and were asked to classify any pain, bleeding, or swelling that had occurred as "none," "mild," "moderate," or "severe."

The findings were quite clear—postextraction complications were reduced significantly by positive suggestion in the waking state and even more so following the induction of a deeply relaxed state. The figure on page 207 is an adaption of the original evaluation sheet for the forty-five people in his study.

No matter how trivial an injury, a tense situation, or a physical symptom, healing is facilitated by focusing the attention on relaxation and an image of health and success. The bricklayer who drops a brick on his foot and goes hopping around on one foot, groaning in pain, is responding maladaptively. He would feel much better if he sat down, relaxed, and imagined rapid healing of his injured foot. He might find that the pain would diminish, swelling would be minimized, and healing would begin immediately and proceed swiftly.

Allowing yourself to begin to relax after an injury or when you begin to experience a familiar symptom is controlling your "fight–flight" responses. If you consciously begin to relax your body, it's a sign to your nonconscious mind that there is nothing to fear, everything is okay, proper treatment will be administered, and there is no danger; the natural healing processes can begin to take over.

Of course, if immediate first aid is necessary such as to control bleeding, this should be done, then followed by a relaxation procedure. Watch your thoughts. Remember, if they are out of proportion to the injury (with a sprained ankle, you might find yourself saying, "Oh, I'll probably be hobbling around for months"), you may slow down the healing processes. A good rule to follow after an injury or at the onset of uncomfortable physical or emotional symptoms is RESTORE RELAXATION AS SOON AS IT IS PRACTICALLY POSSIBLE, You will find that pain and discomfort are reduced and the healing processes are hastened.

13
What you can do now

The fruit

It was reported to the Very Wisest Men of the Land of Fools that the trees were bearing, and so they went out to collect fruit.

The trees, sure enough, were laden, their branches pulled down almost to the ground.

When the Very Wisest Men reached the trees, they fell to discussing which crop they would harvest first. Since they could not come to any agreement on this, they tried another subject. Now they discovered that there was no accord about whether to pluck the fruit with their left or right hands. Then there was another problem of equal difficulty, and another, until they realized that they must withdraw to a more suitable place to thrash things out.

Finally, after full participation of all the learned institutions, all was settled. The Very Wisest Men again found themselves under the trees. But by then it was winter. The fruit had fallen and lay rotting on the ground.

"What a pity that these trees are so treacherous," exclaimed

the Very Wisest Men. "Those branches had no right to swing up again like that. But never mind; you can at least see that the fruit was rotten anyway."

You might be wondering, "How in the presence of acute pain can anybody relax?" You may think that since tension is natural following injury, relaxing in the face of it would require work. This kind of work is the very essence of what we mean when we say it is possible to *control* your own health and well-being. Responses that seem unnatural and difficult become natural and automatic when learned. Remember the example of riding a bicycle for the first time? Once you learn it, it doesn't seem like work at all.

Once you learn the tools, you might find yourself saying after a minor injury, "Of course, I'll relax now—it's natural so my body can heal." While learning, it may seem as though you're fighting a heavy current of thoughts that all say, "This won't work." Be aware that these thoughts may just be your mind throwing old patterns at you, reminding you that since you've never been able to control your own levels of tension before, there's no reason why you should be able to now. Don't worry about these kinds of thoughts. We all have them to some extent. When you pedal a bicycle up to the top of a hill, it may be hard work; but when you reach the top, you can coast down the other side effortlessly.

Expectations

Expectations are thoughts created by the self-image to reinforce your old patterns. Whether your expectations are positive or negative, the nonconscious mind will do its best to make sure that these suggestions are carried out. What will happen to you is often what you now see happening in your imagination. If you were to spend some time each day imagining yourself as you would like to be, your mind would tend to orient you in that direction.

Next time you catch yourself making a mistake, close your eyes for a moment and go through the act again—correctly. Don't just *think* about it; but really *picture* yourself this way, *imagine* how it feels to do it correctly. Imagine it until you really *feel good*. In doing it this way you won't build a habit of making that same mistake over and over. Do you know people who're always losing their keys? Every time they may say, "I always lose them; it's nothing new." The pattern continues to exist in their mind. Perhaps you might suggest a more appropriate comment: "I lost my keys today; next time I'll remember where I put them." Often this simple alteration of expectations will serve to help them break their habit if there are no underlying blocks. Sometimes a habit like always being late or losing keys is a symptom of something deeper. If this is so, an exploration may uncover the underlying roots.

Expectations about the circumstances of our lives can create physical symptoms and maladaptive emotional responses. Imagine the high school girl who is overweight. Her whole family is overweight; she's always *expected* that she would have a weight problem, too, and sure enough, she does. Imagine Bobby, the young boy who had allergies. His mother and father both had allergies when they were young but outgrew them by the time they were twelve. They gave Bobby the expectation—"Don't worry, you'll outgrow them before you go to high school." The summer before Bobby started ninth grade, he noticed that his allergies had disappeared! How many people do you know who say, "I can't sing" or "I can't paint" or "I can't play a musical instrument," because they've built up the expectation that they would fail? Have you ever been around a group of people who have colds and said, "I'll bet I catch one, too," and awakened the next morning with symptoms?

Most of us have grown up with the expectation that when we go to the doctor or dentist we are likely to experience pain and discomfort. It is interesting to observe that this isn't necessarily true. People are now beginning to realize that going to the doctor can be a pleasant, satisfying experience. Learn to have control over your expectations. You'll be surprised at how easy things become.

One example of this is a woman who had been terrified of dentists all her life. She found every aspect of dental work extremely unpleasant. She needed one filling and went into the office nervous and tense. The first thing she told the doctor was that she couldt't stand anyone working on her teeth and she wasn't going to like this at all. The dentist told her that if she would go through a relaxation process, her anxiety would diminish and a new set of expectations could be suggested. She agreed and after about five minutes she was relaxed, and the dentist pressed a probe against her gum. In this way he pretended to give her an injection of novocain while suggesting that she would feel no discomfort. When he had completed filling her tooth, he suggested that she imagine herself feeling good, feeling alert and energetic, and feeling especially comfortable. He also suggested that she feel relaxed and calm about any future dental appointments she might have. She got out of the chair smiling and commented, "I never thought I could actually enjoy the dentist's office!" Later she told the dentist that usually she was unable to eat after dental work, that she frequently vomited and was tense for several days following the appointment. After this appointment she had the urge to go out for dinner and celebrate! All this happened through alterations in her expectations.

Let's look at how the case of a young child—who as yet has few expectations of doctors—illustrates this same point. Perhaps you can use this more positive type of attitude with your own children or children you know.

The "magic spot"

When a young child comes in for treatment, the doctor can take a number of approaches. One choice is: "Well, you've got an infection. We're going to have to give you a shot in your backside and inject this white fluid." Even though the child is promised that it won't hurt any more than a little bee sting, for some reason he doesn't want to sit still. Here's a conversation that demonstrates another way:

DOCTOR: Okay, I've got some "get well medicine" for you.
CHILD: What's that?
DOCTOR: That's a special medicine that helps you get well.
CHILD: What's *well* mean?
DOCTOR: That means you can go out and play tomorrow. Would you like that?
CHILD: Oh, yeah!
DOCTOR: Okay. We're going to give you the medicine in your magic spot; that way you will get well right away.

CHILD: Magic spot?

DOCTOR: Everyone has a magic spot where it doesn't hurt at all, and we can give the medicine that will make them well. Didn't you know that?

CHILD: No! (By this time the child's attention is focused and he can relax.)

DOCTOR: Turn over and I'll show you where it is. Now you help me find the magic spot, okay?

CHILD: Okay!

DOCTOR: Close your eyes, you'll be able to find it better with your eyes closed. It's the spot that feels the most numb. It's right around there, feel it?

CHILD: Uh huh.

DOCTOR: Now, we'll push the medicine right into the magic spot. . . . There you go, all done!

The needle is in, the medicine is administered, the child bounds off the table happily, and that's it. He doesn't feel any pain, he has no expectations of fear, and he is friends with the doctor.

As adults we can easily adjust our expectations if we have negative ones about going to the doctor or dentist. We can recall a few memories of occasions at the doctor's office that were unpleasant and imagine ourselves in the same circumstances but feeling relaxed and comfortable. Through adjusting our self-image, we can change our expectations about the events in our lives.

Do you know of parents who jump every time their child gets a bruise or a scrape? This builds the expectation that anxiety and tension need to be part of every minor injury. What about the parent who says to his or her child, "I'll give you some candy to make the pain go away"? Chances are that this parent will raise a fat child who hasn't learned to deal with pain! And what about the threat, "If you don't behave at the doctor's office, you'll get a shot." This threat of punishment builds up the expectation of fear. When the child really needs a shot, fear will be the primary response.

Instead of saying to a child, "We're going to the doctor to get a shot," it would be much more effective to say, "We're going to the doctor's so you will be more healthy and can play outdoors." "We're going to the dentist to make your teeth strong and white, so you can eat anything you like" is much better than, "We're going to the dentist to have your teeth drilled and filled." Allow the child to explore the clinical environment; he or she will be curious. Allow the child to hold the stethoscope. This will engage the attention and facilitate relaxation instead of creating a fear of a "cold, metal object." As parents begin to understand how expectation can affect experience, so will their children.

What expectations do you have of yourself? Do you expect yourself to always do well? Do you expect that you might fail in spite of hard work? What are your expectations when you are driving the car on the way to the doctor's office? Are you anxious and tense, or are you relaxed? Do you expect that it will be painful? Uncomfortable? Pleasant? What do you expect of your doctor and of the medical profession? Do you worry about your annual checkup? Do you expect that you'll always heal more quickly than average when you take medication? Do you have any expectations about yourself learning relaxation processes? Are they positive? Negative? Realistic? Are you being hard on yourself?

Next time you are on your way to the doctor for an

exam, medication, or for treatment of some sort, spend a few moments imagining yourself feeling calm and relaxed. You are going to the doctor so you can quickly restore balance in your body. The doctor will give you tools to aid your natural healing abilities. Imagine that you feel comfortable talking with the doctor. He or she supports your asking questions and understanding your own symptoms. Your appointment goes smoothly and quickly. When you leave, you feel satisfied that you have taken care of your needs, and you can be free of tension and anxiety.

Wellness—another step

Imagine yourself looking exactly as you would like to look and wearing the clothes you feel especially good in. Imagine that your facial expression says exactly what you'd like to communicate to the people around you. Imagine your body looking exactly as you'd like it to look. Do you feel solid and confident, strong, graceful, relaxed, supple, poised? What thoughts and attitudes would you have if you were your *ideal* self? Imagine yourself going through the day feeling self-assured, energetic, and creative. What would your day be like?

As people alleviate the physical symptoms that cause painful anxiety in their daily lives and establish control of maladaptive tension, many see that the relaxation processes they have learned can be used on a new level—the level of *wellness*.

	0	+
←————————————————	—————————————————→
Disease	Health	Wellness

The health continuum

In our usual medical model, which we can call the "disease-health" model, the physician says to the patient who has become ill, "I will take care of you; give me complete responsibility for your well-being." The patient feels like the unfortunate recipient of a disease from a cruel world, unable to help him- or herself, and subject to the schedule and skill of the physician. If the doctor fails to "cure" the patient, the doctor often feels helpless, perhaps angry at him- or herself and/or at the patient; generally the doctor then refers the patient to a specialist or says to the patient, "I can't make you any better, but I will support you in your helplessness with symptomatic therapy."

In the wellness model, the patient takes responsibility for his/her body, its condition, and his/her health care. If a health problem develops, he/she enlists the aid of the doctor, who gives expert advice. He/she then embarks on a program of rest, exercise, nutrition, and, if necessary, the proper medication after consulting with the physician. He/she also explores the period preceding the illness to find out what was responsible for the drop in resistance, psychological or physical, that allowed the disease state to develop and initiates corrective measures to prevent recurrences. Deep relaxation and image visualizaion are used to diminish symptoms and to promote the healing process. If the disease leaves him/her with some permanent change, imagery is used to integrate this change into the self-image so that she/he is not handicapped by it. As the patient passes from disease through health, she/he gains in self-confidence, becomes more actualized, and has changed his/her life so as to minimize the chances of recurrence of this problem. And the approach that is being used does not stop at health; it propels the patient on to the level of wellness.

Wellness represents the positive end of the health continuum. Each of you has unique natural characteristics and creative talents. Wellness is achieved through the process of becoming aware of your innermost nature and living life according to your natural predispositions. In other words, just as health implies freedom from disease, wellness includes greater creativity in your work and in your hobbies, mastery of your special skills, and fulfillment of your personal desires. Suppose you are a skier or a tennis player. You enjoy the sport but would like to improve your skills. Every time you decide to engage in the activity, you spend five minutes deeply relaxed, imagining yourself as you would like to be, maybe even correcting a weak backhand on the tennis court or an awkward right turn on the slopes. You can become more in harmony with your natural movements and balance and experience more satisfaction from your activities.

As you bring your undesirable patterns to conscious awareness and adjust and expand your self-image to be more adaptive, you may find that the tension and stress that used to be maladaptive can be transformed into creativity energy. Once you resolve the problem of recurrent migraine headaches or an ulcer and have traced these problems to their roots so they are eliminated completely, you may find that you have more energy for other areas of your life. You may want to start a new hobby, increase your skills in a favorite sport or craft, work on better and more effective self-expression, improve your interpersonal relationships, and so on. Using the same tools of relaxation and imagination that helped you eliminate a maladaptive pattern or heal quickly, you can actually expand your self-image to include mastery of the skills you desire and higher levels of creativity.

Let's look briefly at some examples of the use of these tools at the level of wellness. A popular magazine has recently reported that Jean-Claude Killy, Olympic gold medalist, claims that he skied one of his best races after being in a deeply relaxed state and rehearsing the race through his imagination. Albert Einstein discovered and developed the theory of relativity by experiencing internal images in a relaxed state that he then converted to mathematical formulas. In World War II, fighter pilots had to fly continuous missions for many, many hours. While the planes were being prepared on aircraft carriers, the pilots were taken through a progressive relaxation to rest them, so they could stay alert during the long hours in flight.

An experiment was conducted with two groups of people who were interested in learning to increase their reading speed. Each group enrolled in a speed reading course that was to last for ten weeks. One class was told to practice reading techniques for one hour each night. The other class was told to practice the techniques fifteen minutes each night by *imaging* themselves reading. Each group set a reading speed goal for the tenth session. After the fourth session, the people who had been practicing in their imaginations had reached their goals and far surpassed the speed of those tho were practicing one hour a night![1]

A basketball coach was concerned that his team did so poorly at foul shots. He divided the team in half; one-half practiced shooting baskets from the foul line each day, and

[1] Peter H. C. Mutke, M.D., unpublished manuscript, 1970.

the other half rehearsed foul shots in their imagination. This group did so much better after three weeks that the coach decided to end the experiment and have the whole team practice improving their skills in their imaginations while deeply relaxed. Sound unusual? How often have you heard that human beings only use ten percent of their mental capacity? Have you ever wondered about the other ninety percent? Each one of us has tremendous creative potential, and we are just beginning to learn how to train people to tap this vast natural resource.

Select an aspect of your self-image that you'd like to adjust or expand. It may be a physical aspect such as improving your muscle tone, mastering a physical skill, or learning to enjoy the sexual experience more fully; a mental aspect such as reading and studying more or procrastinating less; or an emotional aspect such as becoming more confident, overcoming shyness, or improving interpersonal communication.

In a state of deep relaxation, you can recall a series of memories where this aspect of your self-image that you'd like to strengthen was prominent. As you go through the memories in mental imagery, you get a clear, sensory picture of how your mind and body responded in these situations. Based on the images you recall, you can now improve on the response of your nonconscious mind. You relive the memories, changing your story a bit, adjusting or expanding your behavoir, rewriting your script until you are satisfied with it. You can then project this new, more satisfying behavior onto future situations and imagine yourself as you would like to be.

Here is an example of a young salesman named Ted who wanted to increase his level of self-confidence. Ted's case demonstrates how the use of relaxation and imagination can be applied at the level of wellness. In a state of relaxation, he recalled the following three memories:

> Last week, while making a sale, I felt that I could have sold more and written a larger contract, but I settled for less. I "knew" that a little persistence would have turned a mediocre sale into a real triumph, but I didn't have the courage to try.
>
> A few days ago, my parents said I'd been going out too often in the evenings and should stay home more. I wanted to discuss the fact that I needed a little more freedom in choosing my own life patterns so that I could get out of my unhappy rut, but I've never been able to face up to my parents.
>
> Gloria, my girlfriend, asked the other night if I minded if she had a date with Charlie. I wanted to tell her my true feelings, and I know that it would be possible to express them while still remaining open to her thought, but I was afraid I might say the wrong thing and mess things up. I felt terrible as I told her that I didn't mind.

Next, Ted relived each of these past situations in a state of deep relaxation, imagining himself with the courage to speak his feelings and confront people. He imagined each situation as vividly and as clearly as possible, including the room, the clothes he was wearing, the time of day, where he was sitting, the people in the room and so forth. This time, however, he changed his behavior a bit and rewrote the memories so that things happened the way he wanted. He taught his mind that there were new, creative, and more fulfilling ways of handling his situations. Ted experienced a powerful feeling of triumph when he responded in the desired manner. The emotion of satisfaction was the cue that his mind had accepted the new way of behaving. The deep state of relaxation keeps the mind from its usual automatic responses. When the nonconscious is taught a better, more effective way of responding in a particular situation, it tends to use that new way when a similar situation occurs in the future.

Ted "relived" each of his three memories, adjusting his behavior until he felt the emotion of satisfaction. After reliving them, he imagined similar situations that might occur in the future where his lack of confidence might come up again. He imagined a situation in which Gloria tells him that she's been invited to visit with friends on a night they had planned to go out. She asks him if he would mind if they changed their plans to another night. Ted imagined himself responding, "As a matter of fact, I do mind. I'd really prefer it if *we* went out tonight."

He next imagined that he had an important client who was thinking of shifting his business to a competitor. Ted imagined himself having the confidence to insist that his client give him the opportunity to compare his product with that of the other company and show its advantages, rather than follow his previous pattern of backing down and leaving, empty-handed and dissatisfied. He allowed himself to experience feelings of confidence, pride, and success. He imagined leaving the meeting with a new sales contract in his hand—singing to himself on the way home.

It is important that the goals be kept realistic. There are bound to be many clients who won't be interested in Ted's product. He imagines another situation where a client decides, for realistic reasons, to use a competitor's product. Ted imagines himself doing the best job he can, accepting the choice of his client, and feeling confident about his own skills. How often have you eroded *your* self-confidence by punishing yourself for a "failure" when the circumstances were actually beyond your control?

What is the difference between Ted and the daydreamer who always dreams of success but never achieves it? The daydreamer often uses imagination to *escape* from reality. Ted, on the other hand, was highly motivated and willing to be responsible in choosing realistic alternatives in his self-image. This is the critical difference. While deeply relaxed, attention can be acutely focused on even abstract internal attitudes such as confidence and courage. The daydreamer often doesn't take a responsible attitude that would allow his or her desires to be manifested. He or she wants to be given success and is not willing to put energy behind the image. The nonconscious mind knows whether or not we are serious and willing to work! The daydreamer clings to the self-defeating notion: "If only I could . . . " or "If only I had . . . " Ted didn't want to change the world or the outer circumstances of his life—he wanted to adjust *himself* so that the circumstances he would create would be the ones that fulfilled him and met his needs. The important point is that Ted used a sensitive state of mind to allow him to become more effective in his environment—not to escape from it! Ted's girlfriend, his associates at work, and his parents all began to notice changes in Ted's behavior as Ted himself experienced more self-confidence.

As you think about using these tools for yourself, remember that you can't change other people—you can, however, become more effective in dealing with them. After rewriting your script as described above, it may seem as though the world has changed when actually the change has been in you. Suppose, for instance, that you've had problems with your best friend lately. She has been annoyed with you for having such a pessimistic attitude—everything seems gloomy to you. You've had little energy for social activities, and you've been sluggish at work and at home. You decide to spend some time each day focusing on your positive qualities while relaxed and imagining yourself more enthusiastic and energetic. After several weeks, the problems with your friend have cleared up. In fact, she says she especially enjoys spending time with you now and calls you often. It may appear as though circumstances have changed or your friend has changed. Not so. *You* have! Your self-image has become more adaptive, and your expectations are more positive; so your nonconscious will tend to set up for you the circumstances in your life that fulfill your new self-image.

The time required for each unique individual to adjust an aspect of his or her self-image will vary. It is dependent on your willingness to work, your motivation, and how deeply ingrained the problem is. Perhaps the response you get will be more subtle than you expected. Or maybe your critical factor gets in the way. Maybe you are unrealistic about how you want to expand or adjust your self-image. Will the adjustment conflict with other aspects of your self-image? If you intend to change merely in order to please or impress others, your mind may resist you. Your goal must include a responsible attitude to alter your own patterns. And you must be willing to do without that exquisite pleasure of discouragement and self-pity.

We have seen how relaxation and imagination can be valuable tools for dealing with painful physical and emotional symptoms and maladaptive tension. In addition, they can be used at the level of metahealth to allow you to become more effective and more satisfied in your everyday life. So you see that this newly emerging view of medicine and health covers the entire *health continuum* from disease and cellular dysfunction to joy and creativity. With a new *awareness* of the power you have within to move yourself along the health continuum, you may be beginning to feel changes in your attitudes toward yourself and your own healing abilities even now, at this moment, as you continue to read.

14
The new
"well medicine"

The belly and the other members

It is said that in former times the various members of the human body did not work together as amicably as they do now. On one occasion the members began to be critical of the belly for spending an idle life of luxury while they had to spend all their time laboring for its support and ministering to its wants and pleasures.

The members went so far as to decide to cut off the belly's supplies for the future. The hands were no longer to carry food to the mouth, nor the mouth to receive, nor the teeth to chew it.

But, lo and behold, it was only a short time after they had agreed upon this course of starving the belly into subjection when they all began, one by one, to fail and flop and the whole body to waste away. In the end the members became convinced that the belly also, cumbersome and useless as it seemed, had an important function of its own, and that they could no more exist without it than it could do without them.

APPLICATION: As in the body, so in the state each member in his proper sphere must work for the common good.

The concepts that we've been discussing are part of the frontier of the "new" medicine and are sometimes referred to as *holistic*, *humanistic*, or *patient-oriented* approaches. The trend toward these approaches is becoming more and more apparent in our culture. Perhaps this is the result of the pendulum swinging back from its extreme position in which the physician was given total responsibility for the health of the patient. We have seen how a focus on the psychological aspects of disease combined with the willing participation of the individual has the potential to significantly alter the course of any disease.

This age of specialization and reductionism has produced a philosophy of medicine that is now being challenged. For many years, there has been a growing tendency to view the individual as an aggregate of parts somewhat like a machine or a computer; when one part malfunctions, the patient is referred to an appropriate specialist to have this part repaired. This artificial compartmentalization fails to take into account the ultimate, complicated balance of the *whole* organism.

Many physicians are now taking a new look at the traditional style of medical practice and beginning to see the value of a philosophy that embraces the old view, yet expands it to include a respect for the natural healing capacity of each organism. The following case demonstrates the difference between traditional approaches and the newer, more holistic approaches.

Jane

Jane is a thirty-two-year-old woman who came in for treatment of severe cramps and bleeding between menstrual periods. She was divorced from her husband a year and a half ago, at which time she stopped taking birth control pills and began using an intrauterine device (IUD).

Jane had been forced to stay home from work on many occasions because of the severe cramps, and she was faced with a financial strain in addition to the physical and emotional strain. In order to treat Jane's symptoms, her previous physician decided to remove her IUD and put her back on birth control pills to control the bleeding and cramps. Following the removal of her IUD, she had heavy bleeding for several more days; and her doctor told her to double up on the birth control pills. Symptoms of nausea, bloating, headaches, dizziness, and emotional anxiety followed. Finally Jane underwent surgery to have the lining of her uterus scraped and the tissue examined for abnormalities. Signs of mild hyperplasia (overgrowth of the uterine lining) were found to be the probable cause of Jane's problems. Following surgery, the cramps and bleeding were expected to clear up. They did not.

By this time, Jane had become depressed and discouraged. Her work performance was low and her social and personal life very unsatisfactory to her. She felt she couldn't go on taking birth control pills, even though discontinuing them might result in a worsening of bleeding. Jane talked her problem over with her doctor, and since she felt quite sure that she didn't want to have children, her doctor suggested surgery to remove her uterus.

Jane was frightened by the upcoming surgery. She had had an unpleasant experience with an appendectomy several years before in which she had postoperative complications and a prolonged hospital stay. She came in to explore her fear of surgery and prevent possible complications.

In discussing her history, there was a distinct pattern to the development of her symptoms. We discussed the possible psychological basis of her problems. Jane's marriage had ended because of sexual incompatibility with her husband. She had never been able to fully relax during the sexual experience and had never fully enjoyed intercourse. At the end of her marriage, she was determined to learn more about men and sex. After a series of sexual partners, she still was dissatisfied and unhappy. Her self-confidence continued to drop as she began to doubt whether or not she would ever be able to establish a fulfilling relationship with a man. She soon began to develop cramps immediately following intercourse. She became even more confused and uncomfortable. As her anxiety and tension increased, she began to notice the abnormal bleeding, which contributed even further to her unsatisfactory sexual relationships. The treatment with birth control pills caused a further decline in her self-image and in her willingness to relate to people at work and in social situations.

The spiral continued; anxiety and tension led to cramps and bleeding, which led to more anxiety and tension, which led to worsening of the symptoms, and so on. Jane did not realize that her sexual problems might be responsible for her physical symptoms. In our culture, the doctor's office has not traditionally been a comfortable place to reveal sexual fears and frustrations. The role of emotions and self-image as the root of physical symptoms is seldom given more than lip service by most physicians. A glance at the current statistics concerning hysterectomies supports this. Chances are that significantly fewer hysterectomies would be performed if emotional correlates to the physical symptoms were dealt with. Jane's case is a perfect example.

Jane decided to use an exploration to uncover some of the events that later led her to associate fear and tension with her sexuality. She had grown up with the notion that women should feel guilty if they completely enjoyed the sexual experience (not unlike many other women in our culture). Jane learned the processes of relaxation and began to use them on a daily basis. Slowly her self-image began to adjust itself. After a week, she could feel some changes in her body. The bleeding began to slow down; and after several weeks it stopped, the cramps subsided, and she was having normal menstrual periods. She decided against the surgery.

Jane had adjusted her self-image such that she no longer needed to associate her sexuality and sexual relationships with fear and anxiety. She learned how to control tension in her body so that it didn't become maladaptive. In adjusting her self-image, Jane could see some of the mistakes she had made in her recent relationships and how she had set them up to fail. She learned what "sexual fulfillment" meant to her. Within a few months she had established a satisfying relationship with a man. She had another IUD inserted and used it this time without difficulty.

After several months Jane became engaged and began to consider having children, an option that would have been eliminated had she gone ahead with the scheduled surgery. Now she had the opportunity to experience her life with expanded potential rather than with the limitations that would have been created by the surgery. She had learned tools that allowed her to completely change her life!

It could be argued that the particular doctor was overhasty in scheduling surgery, that the resolution of the problem might have occurred anyway, or that Jane might have discovered a better way of relating sexually on her own. This is, however, but one of many similar cases involving the inattention of the traditional medical model to the psychological and psychosocial aspects of human illness. Of course there are and have been many, many physicians who have been sensitive to these factors and have used the best methods they knew of to help patients resolve them; still, I fear, such doctors are very much in the minority.

Jane's case brings up one of the central differences in point of view between practitioners of the "new" holistic medicine and practitioners of compartmentalized medicine in our culture; this latter attitude is disease and symptom oriented, and often it is crisis oriented. Crisis-oriented medicine means that the symptom or disease is treated only when it becomes a serious problem for the patient—when it becomes painful, debilitating, or causes malfunction of a major organ.

Symptomatic treatment is often prescribed at the expense of uncovering the cause of the problem, thus relieving the immediate crisis of pain, spasm, or malfunction and giving the appearance that the symptom has been cured. If the disease continues despite the covering up of the immediate symptoms, a further search may be necessary, involving X rays, laboratory tests, or perhaps even exploratory surgery. Seldom is much attention paid to the patient's psychological view of what is happening or to his or her need to feel at least in part some control of what's going on rather than just having a sense of being shifted from one laboratory to another. Bills mount up tremendously, and the physical and emotional toll on the patient is high. Months may go by while the patient carries the burden of uncomfortable symptoms with weekly appointments at one laboratory or another for tests to figure out the problem.

If the patient has health insurance, then at least some of the bills are paid. But even this is a mixed blessing. Health insurance plans pay automatically for laboratory work, X rays, many drugs, surgeries, emergency care, hospitalization—all that need be done is to bill them. They will even pay, for instance, for the removal of a small mole that has not shown any malignant potential and has been with the patient all his or her life. In actuality, physicians are rarely, if ever, required to justify these procedures to insurance companies. Unless the doctor is so flagrant in his or her violations as to receive medical censure or to be convicted in a major malpractice suit, he or she may continue to order tests and treatments with abandon, assured that they will be paid for. Often people are admitted to the hospital to have tests that could actually be done in a laboratory, simply because they have only hospitalization insurance. If they had the tests made on the outside, they would have to absorb the financial burden themselves. This whole system leads to an upward climb in medical and laboratory costs and supports the tendency to focus on crisis-oriented medicine.

Paradoxically, many of the same plans that pay thousands of dollars for hospitalization, laboratory tests, and surgery are unwilling to pay for anything at all for three or four treatments designed to teach the patient how to eliminate symptoms before surgery becomes necessary. The exploration of the psychosomatic aspects of disease is often not covered by the same insurance policy unless it covers "psychiatric" treatment.

If a well-meaning physician should charge someone for several hours of instruction in relaxation, imagery, and self-healing, he or she might find an angry patient who insists, "I paid for my insurance; now I want the drugs and treatment it covers." The physician might soon "learn his/her lesson" and limit treatment to the kind that will be paid for, even if it gives only temporary relief. Thus we see a merry-go-round of vastly increasing costs with almost no attention paid to the fact that many people have diseases that could be better approached through enlisting the aid of the patient!

The "patient" in the traditional model of medicine patiently waits for the doctor to do something to relieve a symptom. While physicians' fees mount up, while hospital bills, drugs, and insurance payments accumulate—the patient must sustain losses in freedom, time, self-confidence, and internal control along with the financial strain. The person in the model of the new *well* medicine actively avails him- or herself of the resources that will promote health and well-being, thus adding the educational aspect to the treatment model. The practitioners of holistic medicine *teach* tools that the client can apply before a crisis is reached.

The aim of orthodox medicine as it is practiced in this culture often seems to be to return the patient as closely as possible to a condition where there is "no discernible sickness." Well medicine or holistic medicine takes a broader view. It includes bringing the individual to a state of balance and then on to higher levels of satisfaction, fulfillment, and creativity—*metahealth*. The focus is on the individual and the health of the individual, not on the disease. (It is not uncommon for some physicians to make comments like, "What a day—two cardiac arrests, an appendix, and an overdose," with no mention of the individuals who were the incidental carriers of these problems.) The new frontier in medicine recognizes the importance of the individual, of the quality of her or his life, and of the self-image as essential aspects affecting any medical treatment.

Practitioners of holistic medicine believe that the ideas you put into your mind and the way in which you view yourself and your environment have profound effect on your health and your ability to enjoy life. They support the notion that you are not helpless against a sea of microscopic invaders but that you have a strong connection to your internal defense mechanisms. When you are in a poor emotional or physical balance, your defense mechanisms are not as effective; microorganisms and other invaders may gain the upper hand, just as you are likely to get into more arguments and have more accidents. One purpose of the doctor is to provide access to the skills and tools needed in order to maintain your health and achieve greater satisfaction from life. He or she is committed to developing methods for working with people who are *well*; a greater expenditure on preventive measures can curtail the crises that might otherwise occur.

The placebo effect

The placebo effect demonstrates the significance of expectation in healing. It also shows us the tendency for medical science to sometimes overlook the role of expectation and suggestion as essential components of the healing process. The placebo effect is an improvement in the condition of a patient that occurs in response to treatment but that cannot be considered to be caused by the specific treatment used; rather it is due to the suggestion that the treatment will be effective.

Let's look at an example of how a drug is tested in our culture before it is placed on the market. In a controlled, double-blind study, two groups are tested; each group had the same physical disease. (In a double-blind study, neither patients nor doctors know which group is given the drug or which is given the placebo. This is to prevent their expectations from contaminating the experiment.) The efficiency of the drug is determined by the percentage of cures in the subject groups. Group I receives treatment with the drug, and Group II receives a placebo (an inert and innocuous substance). The results indicate that 60 percent of the patients in Group I responded favorably to the drug.

It would be apparent at first glance that the drug has 60 percent efficacy. But when looking at the placebo group (Group II), it is found that 25 to 30 percent of those patients improved as well. The usual procedure is to subtract the effect of the placebo group from the group given the drug. The results are then stated as follows:

Drug A is twice as effective as a placebo.

Research on the ingredients in the drug would then be continued to strengthen its effect (increase its effectiveness over the placebo).

Practitioners of the new "well medicine" ask, "Why not strengthen the placebo effect?" Since in almost every case there is a distinct percentage of people who improve with just the placebo, why not research the conditions that lead to the placebo effect, strengthen it, and put into practice the fact that a large number of people get better without drugs?

An interesting study similar to the one we just described demonstrates the feasibility of this view. Again Group I was given the drug, and Group II was given a placebo. The results were as follows:

Group I	60 percent of the patients improved
Group II	55 percent of the patients improved

These results seemed especially unusual. All factors were checked, and it was discovered that the doctor who was giving the patients the medications (he didn't know whether he was actually giving the drug or the placebo) was also giving each of them a ten-minute talk on the effectiveness of the medication and telling them they could *expect* very good results! The drug company informed him that he must *stop* giving these positive suggestions so that the actual effectiveness of the drug could be tested.

It's true; the doctor did add another factor to the experiment that made it impossible to determine the actual effectiveness of the drug. But the response of the drug company to discount personal factors and concentrate on "hard facts" represents the attitude taken by many members of the medical profession about the placebo effect. Why not study the group who achieved 55 percent relief without drugs and teach these patients how to use suggestion for themselves or in addition to taking the drug rather than canceling the effect altogether? Imagine the savings in patient costs and drug research.

Before any of these changes can occur, one important criterion must be met—doctors must be able to experience these processes for themselves. They must know that they can control their *own* diseases and that they are effective in doing so. Otherwise, the cues they give patients will be skeptical and unsure rather than confident. Their studies would then "prove" that this approach doesn't work: Suggestions are easily transmitted in subliminal ways both verbally and nonverbally. If the doctors running the experiment are biased against it, most of their patients probably will not respond. Following their study, they would find their beliefs confirmed, that "self-applied healing tools have been shown to function in only a few cases" or "they're not practical." Yet the thousands of people who have experienced these tools for themselves say overwhelmingly, "They work!" We're now in an era where this gap must be resolved, and fortunately, more physicians every day are setting aside their dogma and saying, "I think I'll open up and try it, then judge for myself."

The shift from crisis-oriented medicine to preventive medicine is slow but under way. Every time you or someone you know begins to use these tools, we move another step forward in making medical science more effective for our present-day needs. As we've all heard before, "An ounce of prevention is worth a pound of cure!"

15
The power of the M.D.

The quack frog

A frog, emerging from the mud of the swamp, announced to all the animal world that he could cure every manner of disease. Interested to see what all the croaking was about, the animals gathered around, and the frog, more puffed up than ever by the attention he was receiving, bellowed:

"Here, come and see! You are looking upon the greatest physician in all the world. Not even Aesculapius, Jove's court doctor—"

He was interrupted by a loud bray from the jackass. A goat, also, seemed to be somewhat skeptical of the frog's boastings and said so. Then up spoke the fox: "How dare you set up to heal others? Why do you not try first to cure your own limping gait?"

"And your own bulging and ugly eyes," said the sheep.

At this the quack frog drew in his head and hopped away in the direction of the bog whence he had come while the animals laughed him to scorn.

APPLICATION: Physician, heal thyself!

The old-time family doctor who was characterized by a friendly manner, patience, understanding, and familiarity with the entire family—young and old alike—is rare in our modern culture. In this era of specialization we seldom have a single doctor even for one member of the family. Instead we have several, each with a different area of expertise. As we become more and more removed from a personal doctor–patient relationship, doctors appear more and more powerful and unapproachable. Advanced technology has made doctors gods in the eyes of the public. Modern medicine uses techniques that would stagger anyone's imagination, and doctors alone have the right to use these tools. Because of the power of technology, medical science appears virtually untouchable. What patient would consider visiting his or her doctor to say that the treatment that had been prescribed was inappropriate—that they had discovered a better way?

Medicine has been invested with tremendous fear—doctors fear the crisis of a possible malpractice suit, and patients fear diagnosis of a serious or terminal illness and the financial burden of rising medical costs. Doctors have been given the power to determine life and death. Suppose a patient comes in for treatment of recurring headaches. The doctor tells him that he may have a brain tumor. A physical exam can't demonstrate with certainty that he *doesn't* have a brain tumor, so the doctor orders tests. The patient feels fear, tension, and stress. The doctor must tell the patient all the possibilities; if he doesn't, he can be sued for malpractice. Thus the patient is told he may have a cancer that will kill him, that only the tests can find out, and that the tests may cause chronic headaches, paralysis, meningitis, or sudden death. We have seen from the cases in this book how the nonconscious mind responds to suggestions in the face of tension and stress. Let's look at a dramatic example of this from another culture. The following story was told to me by an army surgeon who had just returned from Africa.

TUMBA

Justice in an African tribe is often swift and harsh. Tumba, a member of the tribe, had committed a serious breach of tribal law and now sat shivering with fear in a circle of grave-faced old men who were elders of the tribe. They were waiting for the witch doctor to ordain Tumba's punishment.

The witch doctor arose and walked over to Tumba, carrying in one hand a small, straw doll dressed to look like Tumba and a broken thigh bone of a chicken in the other. With an air of power and authority, he thrust the bone into the abdomen of the doll, making clear his verdict without a word. The circle of elders arose and left.

Several days later, some workers from the nearby mission hospital found Tumba lying in the weeds on a road leading from his village. He was taken to the hospital and given the usual tests—X rays, a blood count, and a general physical exam. Everything was normal. Yet here was a young man who was strong physically and seemed close to death. Though only partially conscious, Tumba kept repeating the words, "I have sinned, I am cursed, I die!"

The young doctors at the mission hospital insisted that the primitive acts of an African shaman could not override their medical skills. They knew there was no bone in his stomach and devised a plan to change his expectations. They told Tumba that they would operate and remove the bone from his stomach. An injection of thiopental quickly produced a light anesthesia. The doctors made a superficial incision through the outer layers of skin on his abdomen and stitched it up. It appeared as though an actual operation had been performed. When he regained consciousness, Tumba was shown a chicken bone that had ostensibly been removed. Tumba quickly recovered, and in two days he was walking around the hospital and eating normally.

News of Tumba's healing reached the witch doctor! That same night he silently crept into Tumba's hospital room. Tumba was awakened by the soft steps, and when he opened his eyes he saw before him the witch doctor at the foot of his bed, holding the straw doll with the chicken bone still in place!

By morning Tumba could barely move; within twelve hours he was dead. His hospital chart read " . . . death due to cardiovascular collapse of unknown etiology [cause]."

The vast overemphasis on laboratory tests and X rays in our culture, the resulting financial strain on the patient population, and the perversity of "informed consent" (telling the patient of all the possible unpleasant side effects and complications of treatment) is supported by the medical profession by necessity; doctors must practice according to the pattern set by other physicians in the community and protect themselves against malpractice suits. One most unpleasant consequence of this is that the fear, tension, and anxiety created by unpleasant circumstances and the power of the doctor's words may actually cause the symptoms, side effects, and complications that he or she fears the most.[1] Are the suggestions of the doctor in our culture really any less powerful than those of the witch doctor in Tumba's tribe?

Practitioners of traditional medicine may have no knowledge of voodoo curses; yet they may inform patients that they are about to die, impressing on them the belief that the situation is hopeless and that the best that can be done is to relieve the pain and make them as comfortable as possible. It's shocking to think that some diseases or side effects may be the result of a doctor's suggestion that they might occur. Tension, fear, and anxiety may cause the mind to dwell on these suggestions; and before long, symptoms appear. You probably know people who were told they would die or never be able to function normally but who somehow managed to recover far beyond their doctor's expectations. Have you ever wondered how many people like Tumba have instead lived up to the expectation of the all-powerful medicine man? How dare a physician tell a patient with certainty, "You'll never walk again!"?

The sensation of pain renders one especially open to suggestion, both positive and negative. The experience of pain causes the mind to search for an immediate relief. The doctor is in a dilemma. He or she has had no training in medical school to understand these principles. The doctor may not actually understand how powerful his or her words can be. Patients in pain pick up even the most subtle messages from the doctor. They become acutely sensitive to all stimuli in the environment.

[1] See Dr. Barker's study, pp. 206–8.

Looking closely at the statistics, we find that all the technological skills that doctors possess really enable them to treat the actual causes of only a small percentage of all diseases. As we have said, 90 percent of the diseases familiar to us in this culture have psychological components, and medical science can offer only *relief of the symptoms* of these diseases—not the cure.

Let's look more closely at the diseases that have psychological components. In many cases, if patients are motivated, relief of these problems can be achieved by the patients themselves with such methods as the ones we've been discussing.

PAUL

Paul came in for treatment of a "whiplash"; he complained of back and neck pain continuously. His previous treatment had consisted of muscle relaxants, special exercises, and physical therapy.

In an exploration, Paul recalled the details of the accident that caused his back and neck problems. . . . He was just regaining consciousness, lying in the emergency room, terrified to ask about his family who had been in the car with him at the time of the accident. As he was lying there, the doctor touched his neck while he held the X ray up to the light and in a grave tone said, "You're going to have a lot of trouble with your neck."

Later, when Paul and his family were out of the hospital and returning to their normal lifestyle, Paul began noticing the nagging pain and tension in his neck, which seemed to stay the same no matter what he did.

After the exploration Paul realized how the suggestion of a long-term problem in his neck had been built into his expectations following his accident. He had feared a long recovery and was worried about the financial strain on himself and his family if he had to be out of work for a long period. This tension combined with the doctor's unknowing suggestion was enough to cause the symptoms. Paul relived his memory with the new understanding that the doctor was just making a comment about his neck injury, and it didn't necessarily mean that problems would occur. He allowed himself to believe that the doctor, as wise and famous as he was, could be wrong and that he might *not* have a lot of trouble with his neck. In fact, he might surprise the doctor and get well in record time. He was able to restore balance in his neck and back by learning some relaxation processes and using them every day. His symptoms disappeared.

Jackie

Jackie came in for treatment of severe depression. She described herself as "feeling dead—there is nothing living inside." In an exploration she recalled the following memory:

Jackie was in the recovery room following a mastectomy. She was in a semiconscious, highly suggestible state, coming out of the anesthesia. She heard one of the doctors say, "Oh, she has about three years to live."

As it turned out, there was no recurrence of her physical disease; yet we traced an onset of her depression to exactly three years from her surgery! She didn't die physically, but emotionally she no longer felt alive.

Doctors are forced by law to tell all possible side effects of any procedure. But given the vulnerability of the patient in pain, the powerful position of the M.D., and the unawareness of most doctors as to how the mind responds to suggestion under stress, these new tools of holistic medicine are coming at a good time in our culture.

The other side is more optimistic. We can now teach doctors to use the techniques of relaxation and to help patients create positive expectations about their diseases and symptoms along with their regular medical treatment. We can teach them to participate in their own healing processes. We can now begin to sensitize doctors to the importance of subtle, nonverbal cues. There are even ways to get "informed consent" without suggesting disease. We can reallocate some of the funds spent in medical science to teach patients preventive tools. We might be able to decrease some of the need for "rescue teams" of crisis-oriented medicine that cost billions of dollars every year. . . . The potential for better medical care in our culture and for a healthier, more fulfilled population is limitless!

Conclusion

The lioness

A great rivalry existed among the beasts of the forest over which could produce the largest litter. Some shamefacedly admitted having only two, while others boasted proudly of having a dozen.

At last the committee called upon the lioness.

"And to how many cubs do you give birth?" they asked the proud lioness.

"One," she replied sternly, "but that one is a lion!"

APPLICATION: Quality is more important than quantity.

The rapid advances of technology and the race to keep up have created an ethic for many of us that has become deeply ingrained. This great American ethic is famil-

iar to all of us—if a little is good, then *more is better*. More
money, more resources, more defense, more technical de-
velopments, more computers, . . . more relationships,
more education, more opportunities. . . . The list is endless.
Many people are now beginning to realize that we often
abuse life and abuse our most precious gifts. In the quest
for *more*, we often forget that what is most important we
have in abundance—our potential for health, our ability to
love, and our capacity to create and transform experience.

We can observe the effects of the notion, "more is
better," in medicine. We have reached a point, however,
where more medication, more surgery, more therapy,
more specialization, and more technical skills just aren't
enough. These advances are no longer significantly increasing the quality of health care. That's not to say that we
should halt technological development in medicine. But
we can look at progress from a new point of view—as an
expression of creativity rather than from the compulsive
need to get "bigger and better" everything. Can you *feel*
the difference in the levels of tension associated with those
two perspectives?

We're in an era that's calling for balance—balance in
the social structure, balance in the environment, balance in
the family unit, and balance within each individual. There
is a newly emerging priority for self-control and self-
responsibility that leads to the fulfillment that comes out of
freedom rather than dependency.

It takes courage to be a pioneer. Many of our greatest
scientists and creative artists were scoffed at because of
their innovative notions. Only years later were their insights appreciated. As Abraham Maslow once noted about
creative insight:

> In the early stages of any inquiry it is a mistake to lay down

a hard-and-fast distinction between a scientific investigation of the facts and philosophical reflection about
them. . . . At the later stages the distinction is right and
proper. But if it is drawn too soon and too rigorously those
later stages will never be reached.[1]

It is possible to *know* and *experience* the complexity of the
human mind long before we have scientific evidence to
prove our experience. The changes in the institution of
medical science will come about through the experiences
and support of pioneers of the new medicine—people like
yourself who are willing to explore the limits of the accepted body of knowledge and move the frontier forward
toward better health for our population.

Each of us has new options, new opportunities, new
challenges, and new risks to face. You might imagine that
your body is like a beautiful musical instrument. You can
play vibrant, harmonious music with your instrument; you
can also make noise. Your instrument must be finely
tuned; tonal discord causes displeasure, anxiety, and dysfunction. Even if you are truly a master at playing your
instrument, the sound will not be pleasant and satisfying if
it is improperly tuned. However, when your instrument is
tuned up and played with ease, there is a particular, indescribable quality that you can *feel*. It can't be explained—it
must be experienced. Can fulfillment, pleasure, or really
feeling good ever be described in words? So it is with the
healing processes we've discussed throughout this book.
Explanation can offer you new options, new insights, and
new awarenesses; yet most importantly, the final *experience*
of it all is uniquely yours.

[1]Abraham Maslow, *Towards the Psychology of Being*, New York: Van
Nostrand Reinhold Company, 1968, Foreword.

Appendix

Self-Imagery Cassettes by Dr. Miller

Now you have the opportunity for Dr. Miller's personal guidance:

Each of us, whether we are awake or asleep, is continuously recording "mental videotapes" and storing them with a selectivity and speed of retrieval that staggers the imagination. These stored images are the models upon which all our actions and reactions are based.

The essence of Dr. Miller's work is the study of the nature of these "mental videotapes," or images, to determine which are most regularly associated with good health, high-level wellness, and optimal performance.

The tapes listed below present these images, or "programs," through the medium of audio and video cassettes. The **Selective Awareness** state of deep relaxation is often used to increase the depth of penetration of these models and to provide ongoing stress reduction. Further, it provides a calm space in which to access one's deeper values and personal mission. The resulting self-healing, inspiration, enthusiasm, and sense of wholeness are then integrated into one's mental, emotional and physical life through effective, yet simple, visioning techniques.

The lapping waves of the Carribean Sea, birds from mountain meadows and other nature sounds, along with sensorily rich music and visual images, are used to maximize enjoyment of use.

Dr. Miller offers a set of highly enjoyable, easy to use, programs.

To learn and apply the material presented in this book on a deeper, experiential level, Dr. Miller suggests you begin with one or more of the following programs:

Healing Journey (#16), Letting Go of Stress (#23), Writing Your Own Script (#202), Health and Wellness (#18), Ten-Minute Stress Manager (#53), or

select one of the programs which focuses on a specific problem you may have. Complete instructions for use of all tapes are included with each program.

TO ORDER, OR FOR MORE INFORMATION ABOUT DR. MILLER'S WORK, WRITE OR CALL:

Source Cassettes
P.O. Box W, Dept. 601
Stanford California, 94305
(415)-328-7171 - For Information and California Orders
1-(800)-52-TAPES - For Orders Only (outside California)

Sampler cassette of Emmett Miller programs available for $2.00 redeemable with next order.

EXPERIENTIAL AUDIO CASSETTE LISTING

STRESS MANAGEMENT

LETTING GO OF STRESS. This program teaches a logical progression from simple to sophisticated techniques for stress management. It includes methods to help relieve anxiety, tension, and the physical symptoms of stress. #23. $10.95

THE TEN-MINUTE STRESS MANAGER. Each ten-minute experience is a quick battery charge for executives, students, managers and homemakers. #53. $10.95

THE SOURCE MEDITATION. "Opening Gates to Universal Energy - Life, Breath, Creativity, Wisdom." Provides meditations based on Yogic, Zen Buddhist, and other approaches. #42. $10.95

EASING INTO SLEEP. Those who have used it call this tape "the closest thing to a cure for insomnia." Experience a process that melts away restlessness and leads to deep sleep. #20. $10.95

RAINBOW BUTTERFLY. To enhance and deepen meditative skill, to help improve a bad day or lighten a mood. Journey through the color spectrum, and the metamorphosis of a butterfly. Help color your future bright and beautiful. #11. $10.95

BEHAVIOR CHANGE

TOOLS FOR TAKING CHARGE. An introduction to techniques of managing stress energy through deep relaxation, meditation, autogenic training, guided imagery, and selective awareness (no music). #10. $10.95

WRITING YOUR OWN SCRIPT. Eliminate unwanted attitudes, emotions and habits by replacing negative self-images with exciting new self-concepts for the future. #202. Two Cassettes. $15.95.

SMOKE NO MORE. Quit or cut down using the simple process that replaces the false relaxation of smoking with techniques for utilizing natural stress energy to create the self-image of a healthy non-smoker. #221. Two Cassettes. $15.95

IMAGINE YOURSELF SLIM. This program treats overweight as a symptom, not a cause, and promotes change of self-image and eating habits. Learn to eat only what you need, independent of emotional triggers. #19. $10.95

SEXUAL INTIMACY: RELAXATION AND IMAGERY TO ENRICH THE EXPERIENCE OF MAKING LOVE. The experience of making love can be more than merely physical. It can be a richly rewarding emotional, mental and even spiritual experience. The experience of this kind of sexual intimacy can only be described as magic. Listen -- experience it yourself and with a loved one. #52.
                                                          $10.95

ACCEPTING CHANGE, MOVING ON. Changes in life, in a relationship -- separation, or even death -- can be met with acceptance and experienced as positive challenges. You are guided through the process of putting the past to rest and awakening to a brighter future. #48. $10.95

FREEING YOURSELF FROM FEAR. Fear is the greatest obstacle to personal progress. Some people fear rejection or failure. Some have phobias about people or situations. This program is an antidote for fear, utilizing a powerful step-by-step approach to ensure victory over potentially threatening situations. #338. Three Cassettes. $27.50

BLOSSOMING, GROWING BEYOND THE LIMITS OF YOUR FAMILY. Designed to help adult children of alcoholics lead more satisfying and productive lives. Developed in conjunction with family therapist, David Shearer, this series of eight experiences, selected from Dr. Miller's self-imagery programs, helps to correct the negative impact of growing up in an alcoholic home. This program helps reshape the negative thoughts, attitudes, reactions, feelings and self-image. It teaches deep relaxation skills for stress reduction, relaxation, self-enhancement and visualization skills for using imagery effectively to produce feelings of peace and trust in oneself. #400. Four Cassettes.
                                                          $37.50

PEAK PERFORMANCE

OPTIMAL PERFORMANCE, REACH FOR YOUR GOAL. "Go for the Gold!" Whatever your job, profession, hobby, sport or activity -- this cassette can help you become a winner. Learn how champions reach their goals -- and how you can do the same. An exciting motivational experience for those who strive for excellence. #54. $10.95

YOU DESERVE TO BE RICH. "The Inner Path to Wealth." Become attuned to your deeper values and discover your personal mission. Commit to honest sharing and true wealth will flow to you. Deprogram negative attitudes about money and create a prosperous self-image. #50. $10.95

HEALING THE PLANET. The time is right to share a global vision. Words and music combine for a beautiful, inspiring look at our potential as a global human family. On Side Two, a meditation on love as the source of peace. #101. $10.95

WINNING AT LEARNING. Accelerated learning, peak performance, test-taking skills and stress reduction. This program offers powerful aids for those endeavors where retention and retrieval of information is vital -- school, business, sports, acting, public speaking. #207. Two Cassettes. $15.95

HIGH PERFORMANCE SPORTS. Techniques for using stress energy to achieve your optimal performance. Learn focused concentration and guided imagery skills. Used by competitive and recreational athletes. #228. Two Cassettes. $15.95

HEALTH & SELF-CARE

LETTING GO OF DIS-EASE. An interview with Dr. Miller by Michael Toms of New Dimension magazine on the meaning of healing and the body as a "symptom." #ND-1. $10.95

DOWN WITH HIGH BLOOD PRESSURE. Powerful drug-free techniques for controlling high blood pressure. Clinically proven. Change your reaction to life's stressors. #03. $10.95

HEALING YOUR BACK. Four parts -- Music and imagery to relax away pain and tension; tracing your symptoms to their source; special morning and evening experiences to keep you well. #05. $10.95

GREAT EXPECTATIONS. "The Joy of Pregnancy and Birthing with Techniques for an Easy Delivery." A loving guide through pregnancy. Consistent with Lamaze and other childbirth methods. #30. $10.95

HEADACHE RELIEF. Powerful techniques for headache relief through tension reduction methods with morning and evening exercises. #12. $10.95

AN ANSWER TO CANCER. Based on his work with patients as medical director of the Cancer Support and Education Center, Dr. Miller has created a special version of his widely acclaimed Healing Journey cassette. Side One features the popular "Healing Image." Side Two features "Targeting Your Treatment," which presents special imagery for cancer patients as an adjunct to medical treatment. #29. $10.95

AWAKENING THE HEALER WITHIN -- 1986 Lectures at the Cancer Support & Education Center. Dr. Miller shares his twenty years of clinical experience supported by the latest research in psychoneuroimmunology. Topics include the power of awareness and attitude, healing imagery, self-expression and the immune system, and the role of faith. #229. $15.95

HEALING JOURNEY. Learn techniques for active participation in your body's healing process, especially valuable for acute or chronic conditions. #1 $10.95

SUCCESSFUL SURGERY AND RECOVERY. Condition the mind and body to achieve maximum benefit and speedy recovery from surgery. Techniques to minimize anethesia, post-operative swelling, pain, bleeding and infection. #203. Two Cassettes. $15.95.

HEALTH AND WELLNESS. Techniques for reaching high levels of wellness including personal approaches to diet, exercise, motivation and stress management. Restore balance to your life. #18. $10.95

CHANGE THE CHANNEL ON PAIN. "Managing Pain Successfully." Your mind receives pain messages much like a TV receives a broadcast signal. Using this tape, those with occasional or chronic pain can learn to "change the channel," tune out pain and tune in relief. #46. $10.95

SPECIAL PROGRAMS

SELF-HYPNOSIS AND PERSONAL DEVELOPMENT. Recorded live at the University of California, Berkeley, this has been acclaimed the finest course on the use of self-hypnosis for personal growth offered anywhere. A lively, enjoyable program in which the humor, student participation and fun have been carefully preserved. Techniques for stress reduction, imagery, using disease as a teacher, neutralizing fear, phobias, and other negative feelings, overcoming obstacles to personal development, cultivating a positive self-image and writing your own script. #803. Eight Cassettes in a custom case.
                                                $59.95

RIGHT IMAGERY - WISDOM OF THE EAST AS A BASIS FOR HEALING IMAGERY. Dr. Miller's keynote address to an audience of physicians and other health professionals at the Second International Conference on Eastern and Western Approaches to Healing. He shares his experiences of Eastern disciplines with their focus on "being" with the Western emphasis on "doing," which is a fundamental cause of stress. #CL-1. $10.95

EXPERIENTIAL VIDEOS - A Totally New Concept.

A beautiful sequence of visual images has been developed with the award winning cinematographer -- Glen Carroll.

Dr. Miller's soothing voice and a stereophonic high fidelity soundtrack welcome the viewer to a gently flowing montage of nature images ... rippling streams, crashing surf, golden hills and peaceful sunsets. This sequence, "Watervisions," provides the visual portion of the following video cassettes. Each contains skillfully chosen narration to create the inner experience suggested by each title. Available in VHS, Beta and 3/4" formats.

RELAXATION AND INSPIRATION. Discover how quickly you can let go of stress. Dr. Miller guides you to a deeper inner awareness of peace, inspiration, power and healing. Excellent for a 15 minute midday mini vacation, or use the entire 25 minutes (the final 10 minutes features gentle music and visuals only) to unwind at the end of a busy day. Soothing both as a participatory experience, and as a background piece that turns your television into a work of art. #944 - 25 min. $49.00

STRESSBREAK. In less time than the average coffee break, you can help your employees dramatically reduce tension and prevent stress overload. They will become aware of and focus on the current goal or project and mentally rehearse individual and team optimal performance. #941 - 13 min. $139.00

A TIME TO HEAL. Imagery experiences to enhance the healing response. It is perfect for use in clinics, professional offices, for shut-ins and in hospitals. Closed circuit or individual floor application helps patients adjust, reduce pain and fall asleep with a minimum of medication and nursing care. #942 - 25 min. $89.00

SERENITY. This teaches techniques for relaxing without chemicals. Using relaxation, imagery and affirmations based on the time-tested twelve steps, this program is valuable during withdrawal and to prevent relapses. It is used for alcoholism and drug rehabilitation. #943 - 25 min. $89.00

Bibliography

Part I

A.—The following books are entertaining, fast reading books that give a general overview of the problem engendered by the fact that we must struggle with the curious combination of an ancient, animallike body and subconscious mind with a socialized, civilized, conscious one.

> *Man's Presumptuous Brain: An Evolutionary Interpretation of Psychosomatic Disease,* Simeons, Albert T. Dutton (New York: 1961).
>
> *The Naked Ape,* Morris, Desmond (New York: Dell, 1969).

B.—The relationship between stress and physical disease was first developed by Hans Selye, who coined the word "stress." His book on the subject is:

> *Stress of Life,* Selye, Hans (New York: McGraw-Hill, 1956).

C.—A book for both health professionals and lay readers:

Mind As Healer, Mind As Slayer, Pelletier, Ken (New York: Delta, 1977).

Dr. Pelletier provides an excellent overview of recent research findings, relating stress, personality, lifestyle, and physical disease. He also discusses several methods of relaxation and imagery and the experimental results of their application in clinical settings.

D.—Many texts have appeared during recent years that are quite effective in helping individuals to relax and develop imagery and learn that state of mind that seems to promote balance and health.

Be Here Now, Baba Ram Dass (New York: Harmony, 1971).

Relax—How You Can Feel Better, Fadiman, Jim and John White (New York: Dell, 1976).

Relaxation Response, Benson, Herbert, and Miriam Z. Klipper (New York: Avon, 1976).

Well-Body Book, Samuels, Mike and Hal Bennett. (New York: Bookworks, 1973).

Part II

A. — For the professional who wishes to learn more about relaxation, hypnosis, and the like, I recommend:

> "Findings in Hypnosis," Elman, David, available from Colleen R. Elman, 56 Edgewood Avenue, Clifton, New Jersey, 07012.

This text was written by the late David Elman, who as a lay hypnotist taught many physicians throughout the country to use what was then a nearly unknown tool.

B. — An excellent basic text on hypnosis and hypnotherapy:

> *Clinical and Experimental Hypnosis,* Kroger, William (Philadelphia, PA: Lippincott, 1963).

Details are given clearly enough so that a physician or therapist can begin to use hypnosis almost immediately. Application to surgery, obstetrics, wound healing, anesthesia, phobia deconditioning, and so on are outlined clearly. I highly recommend this book.

C. — Another excellent text on hypnosis which focuses on the development of a systematic approach to hypnotherapy, is:

> *A System of Medical Hypnosis,* Meares, Ainslie (Philadelphia, PA: Saunders, 1960).

D. — An excellent exposition of the practical, theoretical, and experimental bases for many of the techniques used in approaches such as the selective awareness exploration can be found in:

> *Psychotherapy by Reciprocal Inhibition,* Wolpe, J. (Stanford, CA: Stanford University Press, 1958).
>
> *Hypnotic Realities: The Induction of Clinical Hypnosis & Forms of Indirect Suggestion,* Erickson, Milton (New York: Irvington, 1976).

E. — The following text presents an intriguing holographic model for memory storage and retrieval which is highly consistent with the method and findings of the selective awareness exploration

Languages of the Brain, Pribram, K. (Englewood Cliffs, N.J.: Prentice-Hall, Inc., 1971).

Part III
A book which is a perennial favorite and gives a good basic approach to the concepts of self-image building:

Psycho-Cybernetics, Maltz, Maxwell (North Hollywood, CA: Willshire Book Company, 1969).

Additional References

Brallier, Lynn. *Successfully Managing Stress.* (National Nursing Review.)

Dossey, Larry. *Beyond Illness.* (Boston: Shambhala, 1984). and *Time, Space and Medicine.* (Boston: Shambhala, 1982).

Jaffe, Dennis. *Healing From Within.* (New York: Knopf, 1979).

Sheikh, Anees A., (ed.). *Imagery: Current Theory, Research and Application.* (New York: John Wiley & Sons, 1982).

Simonton, Carl S. Matthews-Simonton, and J. Achterberg. *Getting Well Again.* (Los Angeles: J.P. Tarcher, Inc., 1978).

Index

A

Abdomen, gridiron syndrome, 160
Acne, case history, 100
Adrenalin, 152
Advertising
 resistance to, 132
 and self-image, 95
Alcohol, 110–11
Allergies, 147–51
 and expectation, 212–13
Ambiguity, 93
Amputation, case history, 163–64
Analysis, and critical thinking, 27–29

Angina pectoris, 50
 case history, 169–70
Antibiotics, 81–82
Antihistamines, 147, 149
Antihypertensive drugs, 53
 and n.
Anxiety. *See also* tension; stress
 generalized, 134
 maladaptive habits, 110–11
 physical symptoms, 37–57
Appendicitis, 49
Arthritis
 and stress, 168
 used to manipulate others, 189
Asthma
 and muscle spasm, 46–48

The Personal Consultant Newsletter

Thanks to your many requests, I am now publishing a newsletter that will be of real use to you in achieving your maximum personal potential, in both your work and daily life, *The Personal Consultant Newsletter*.

Achieving your optimal potential has always been one of the key purposes of my cassettes and lectures. Through this newsletter you'll receive the latest in concepts, choices, and resources that can make a real difference in how you feel and increase your level of performance and success.

Consider my newsletter to be a tool—a resource for you to use in your personal growth.

Each issue contains my Editorial, along with the Resources Column, Calendar of Events, Question & Answer "Reader's Forum," News & Reviews, "Personal-Performance," How-to Articles and the latest in Medical News and Reviews, to help you do your best.

Take just a minute out of your busy life and write me for subscription information.

Emmett Miller, M.D.
Personal Consultant Newsletter
P.O. Box W
Stanford, California 94305
or Call (415) 328-7171

A WORD FROM THE PUBLISHER

Celestial Arts is the publisher of many excellent books on health and wellness, with an emphasis on topics of awareness such as rebirthing, meditation, consciousness, and miracles.

Among our finest publications are Bob Mandel's *Open Heart Therapy*, Richard Moss's *How Shall I Live*, and Kenneth Pelletier's *Towards A Science of Consciousness*.

We also publish the bestselling books by Sondra Ray, Virginia Satir, Jerry Jampolsky, and Barry Stevens.

For a complete list of our books, please write for our free catalog or call us.

Celestial Arts
P. O. Box 7327
Berkeley, California 94707
(415) 524-1801

A WORD FROM TEN SPEED PRESS

In 1983, *Celestial Arts* joined the publication program of the publishing house *Ten Speed Press*. *Ten Speed's* list includes career and life guidance books, fine cookbooks, bicycling, outdoors, and historical reprints. Please write for their free catalog: *Ten Speed Press, P. O. Box 7123, Berkeley, California, 94707 (415) 845-8414.*

ISBN: 0-89087-458-1 $8.95

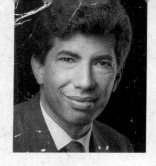

- *Learn how to change unwanted behavior patterns—stop smoking, lose weight*
- *Understand how your self image effects your health*
- *Find the inner path to success and personal fulfillment*

Emmett Miller is a physician, mathematician, musician and poet who has won international acclaim as a pioneer in Humanistic Psychology and the emerging "New Medicine."

Dr. Miller's instruments are not scalpels and drugs, but words and experiences... images and memories...techniques which teach people to relax and inspire them to take charge of their lives and realize their full potential.

He currently resides in the Stanford area of California where he practices his subspecialty of psychophysiological medicine, the use of self care approaches to create balance and health among the mental, physical, emotional and spiritual aspects of human life.

Throughout *SELF IMAGERY*, the emphasis is upon enhancing an individual's innate capacity to attain and maintain health. After many years in medical practice, Emmett E. Miller has modified clinical hypnosis, relaxation methods, and imagery approaches into the comprehensive systems of "Selective Awareness." Using numerous case examples as well as familiar fables, the practice of selective awareness is brought to bear upon the common disorders of headaches, asthma, gastrointestinal tract problems, muscle spasms, circulatory disorders, sexual dysfunction, and a vast range of psychosomatic disorders. One of the most striking aspects of the book is that the method of presentation is consistent with the content since the reader is guided through a progressive series of relaxation and visualization exercises. Most importantly, Miller emphasizes that these approaches are not a panacea and the result is an effective, professional and balanced perspective from a skilled clinician.

> *Kenneth R. Pelletier, Ph.D.*
> *Assistant Clinical Professor,*
> *Dept. of Medicine,*
> *University of California, San Francisco*

Dr. Emmett Miller has distinguished himself as one of the leading theoreticians and practitioners in the emerging era of health care. This book is a model of clarity and usefulness, and will be of enormous help to anyone who senses the role of consciousness in health.

> *Larry Dossey, M.D.*
> *Dallas Diagnostic Association*

To feel good is to live our human heritage. Dr. Emmett Miller shows us how to do this.

> *Virginia Satir, ACSW*
> *Director of Training, Avanta Network*

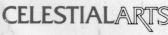

CELESTIAL ARTS

Berkeley, California